Changing practices in primary care

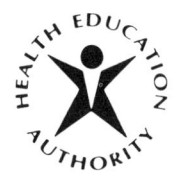

Changing practices in primary care

A facilitator's handbook

ALISON WILSON

Formerly Northern Facilitator Training Officer
National Facilitator Development Project

ISBN 0 7521 0060 2

© Health Education Authority, 1994
First published 1994
Health Education Authority
Hamilton House
Mabledon Place
London
WCIH 9TX

Cover picture reproduced by kind permission of Barnaby's Picture Library

Printed in Great Britain by Bell and Bain Ltd., Glasgow

Contents

Preface

This handbook aims to support the growing numbers of professionals and lay people who are involved in facilitating change in primary care.

It is intended to provide an introduction to facilitation and development of primary care and to be used as an easy reference, for particular aspects of the facilitator's role. Background information is included on general practitioner's services; quality and medical audit; disease and health promotion; an introduction to the role of the primary care facilitator, and the skills facilitators use to encourage the development of primary care services.

A list of abbreviations used in the text appears at the beginning of the book and a bibliography and an extended list of further reading and resources at the end.

The handbook is not intended to replace relevant training and experience, and much of the subject matter is covered in depth in the facilitator training courses organised by the NFDP. The section on health promotion is necessarily only a basic theoretical overview. Health promotion in primary care most often takes the form of short interventions with clients attending the practice. Interviews of this kind require special skills to make the short encounters effective. The HEA therefore, has developed a course to teach facilitators how to prepare health promotion nurses to help clients make changes in health behaviour. These courses, known as 'Helping People Change', are supported by a training manual which supplements this handbook.

The contents have been widely researched, and experienced facilitators working in the field have been extensively consulted on the relevance and accuracy of the material. Primary care is, however, a changing world, and although from time to time different issues or topics assume greater importance, the skills needed to promote or manage change are enduring.

Communication and collaboration between primary care and other organisations, is now more important than ever before. This handbook is therefore likely to have wide appeal and applicability for those embarking on joint projects with the primary care sector and will be a useful introduction to primary care for medical and nursing students on community attachments, GP trainees and newly recruited practice staff.

Acknowledgements

There are a great many people to whom I am indebted for giving help, advice and encouragement whilst writing this book. These include:

- All primary care facilitators who in spring 1991 completed the extensive questionnaire used to establish the main subject areas and special skill needs of facilitators.

- Caroline Hawkridge and Jill Spratley for the initial advice on writing this text.

- Critical readers Hillary Fender, Claire Lloyd, Fiona Young, Margaret Gosling, John Hooker, Lesley Wimpenny, Elaine Fullard and Tony Dowell, who gave their expert advice on the relevance, accuracy and readability of the handbook.

- The facilitators attending Induction courses in 1992/3, and Dr Godfrey Fowler OBE, Dr J A Muir Gray and Mary Blackall, for their advice and encouragement and for their comments and suggestions for improvements.

- The authors of the numerous texts from which I have drawn the material on which to base this handbook.

- The HEA and in particular Dr Jennifer Newton who provided the funding to produce the handbook.

Very special thanks are also extended to Elaine Fullard and Tony Dowell who have provided constant help, encouragement and critical assessment throughout the numerous drafts and redrafts, and to Joy Rayner who has courageously plodded on with the laborious task of typing and retyping the text throughout its various stages.

Abbreviations

APCF	Association of Primary Care Facilitators
BMA	British Medical Association
CHC	Community Health Council
CHD	Coronary heart disease
DHA	District health authority
DOH	Department of Health
FHSA	Family Health Service Authorities
FPC	Family Practitioner Committee
GMSC	General Medical Services Committee
GP	General practitioner
HA	Health authority
HDL	High density lipoprotein
HEA	Health Education Authority
HE(P)O	Health education (promotion) officer
HNA	Health needs assessment
IPR	Individual performance review
LDL	Low density lipoprotein
LMC	Local medical committee
LOT	Local organising teams
MAAG	Medical Audit Advisory Group
MI	Myocardial infarction
NFDP	National Facilitator Development Project
NHS	National Health Service
NHSME	National Health Service management executive
OPCS	Office of Population Census and Surveys
PACT	Prescribing analysis and cost data
PGEA	Postgraduate education allowance
PRP	Performance related pay
RHA	Regional health authority
RCGP	Royal College of General Practitioners
SMR	Standardised mortality ratio
TC	Total cholesterol

1 Working in primary care

The development of primary care and the changes in the NHS

The most significant developments within general practice since 1948 have been the *Charter for the Family Doctor Service* (Department of Health and Social Security, 1965), *Promoting Better Health* (Secretary of State for Social Services, 1987), *Caring for People* (Secretary of State for Health, 1989a), *Working for Patients* (Secretary of State for Health, 1989b), GP Contract (April 1990) and the *Patient's Charter* (Deparment of Health, 1992a).

CHARTER FOR THE FAMILY DOCTOR SERVICE

This Charter took place at a time of great disorder and lethargy within general practice and was the result of direct action from the profession itself. It was constructed by the GMSC of the BMA and served to form the basis of a new contract.

Following its acceptance by the government, profound changes were made in practice structure. Competition was largely removed, assistance provided for obtaining appropriate premises, postgraduate education was supported and the employment of practice ancillary staff facilitated. The Charter also called for a reduction in list sizes and established different methods of payment.

An era of improved morale followed and this led to increased recruitment to general practice. Although the Royal Commission on the NHS in 1979 set out broad objectives for general practice including the patient's right to consult a doctor, change practitioner and choose a hospital with the help of the GP, little was offered to clearly define the exact role of general practice.

PROMOTING BETTER HEALTH

In 1987, following a period of consultation on the government's proposals for changes in primary health care, the White Paper *Promoting Better Health* was published.

The main aims were to:

● Introduce new contracts to doctors and dentists.

- Raise standards of care.
- Place more emphasis on health promotion and disease prevention.
- Provide patients with more information and choice.

Further reforms have evolved from *Promoting Better Health*.

WORKING FOR PATIENTS

This is mainly concerned with the management and funding of the NHS (largely reinforcing *Promoting Better Health*). The proposed changes are aimed at increasing efficiency and making services more responsive to their users through the introduction of new management arrangements.

Changes in management structures and allocation of resources

Working for Patients introduced the notion of 'purchasers' of NHS services and 'providers' of care. The government proposed this separation of funding and the provision of services in order to bring about improvements in the quality and efficiency of services. This is brought about by providers having to compete for business.

The function of the DHA under this new system is to:

- Assess and determine the health needs of its population.
- Purchase, on behalf of its population, services to meet those needs.

The DHA, therefore, takes on a purchaser role. The HA receives funds in order to purchase services for their population instead of beig allocated funds to provide services in their hospitals. Allocations are made on a weighted capitation basis. The DHA then negotiates contracts with providers. The money then follows the patient (even if that means the service is provided outside the district). Likewise GPs who become fund holders will also become purchasers of hospital and eventually community services. GPs who are eligible, receive a practice fund or budget from the RHA to buy a defined range of services for their patients and to cover prescribing costs. FHSAs monitor the expenditure of GPs and continue to allocate development funds for practice staff and premises. (All practices now receive an indicative prescribing budget which is monitored by the FHSA.) The amount of money allocated to GP fundholding practices is deducted from the DHA purchasing funds.

The responsibility of providing services rests with hospital and other 'provider' units, for example health promotion units, community nursing units or private sector health care. Some of these units and hospitals may become NHS Trusts. Although given a great deal of autonomy to manage their hospital or unit, trusts are directly responsible to the Secretary of State. These 'self governing' units which are run by a board of directors, are free to determine their own management structure, employ their own staff (negotiating local pay and conditions) and are free to borrow to develop services or retain any surpluses. The trust must however submit an annual business plan for approval by the NHSME and must publish an annual report and accounts.

Trusts need to win contracts to provide services required by DHAs, GP fundholders and other possible purchasers in order to generate income. This incentive system is therefore intended to ensure quality of service improvements for patients.

In some areas, purchasing authorities or consortiums, who represent DHAs and FHSAs and include specialist advisors, have been set up to take over the sole purchasing role of the DHAs.

Managing clinical activity

Working for Patients builds on the recommendations of the Griffiths Report (Department of Health and Social Security, 1983) which introduced general managers at region, district and unit levels, who are responsible for the performance of their organisation. Part of that management role included resource management initiatives. This initiative has led to the introduction of:

● PACT data to monitor prescribing patterns.
● Medical advisor appointments to FHSAs to review clinical issues with GPs, e.g. referral patterns and PACT data.
● Medical audit in hospitals and primary care, to ensure clinical practice is reviewed and to identify areas where improvements can be made.

Managers are also now involved in the appointment of consultants and undertaking their performance reviews.

CARING FOR PEOPLE

Gives local authorities the lead responsibility in planning and co-ordinating the provision of community care. Community care plans are developed with NHS authorities and other providers of care. Although many of the services are currently provided directly by the local authorities their role will increasingly become that of purchasers, co-ordinators and monitors of the quality of care in the community.

Collaboration between local authorities, DHAs and FHSAs

underpin the success of this initiative. It is hoped that the result will be a more fully integrated service for clients and their carers and will lead to more effective targeting of resources.

THE GP CONTRACT

See section 'The GP contract' page 11.

THE PATIENT'S CHARTER

This forms the response by the NHS to the *Citizen's Charter* which came into operation in 1991. The emphasis of the *Citizen's Charter* is to empower citizens and make public services take consumer wishes into account in providing services. Its main themes include improving quality, giving more choice and setting minimum standards, whilst ensuring value for money.

The *Patient's Charter* came into operation in 1992 for secondary care and in 1993 for primary care. All HAs have been expected to develop and publish their own local charters, which should cover their population's needs. FHSAs have the additional task of encouraging and supporting practiced-based Charters.

CONCLUSION

Changes in the NHS are occurring at a rapid pace. Although overall aims have been set out in the various white papers, their implementation has been left to local interpretation.

Facilitators should be aware of the overall principles of the latest reforms but will need to investigate how these reforms affect the local community in which they work. For example, in some areas the level of GP fundholding remains low and so the impact of fundholding on service provision is likely to be minimal. Each year new 'waves' of practices are likely to become eligible for fundholding status. The effects of full market forces are not yet known as practices have been restricted from 'freely' placing their contracts where they would like.

FHSAs, DHAs and public health departments are faced with the challenge of defining health needs and ensuring those needs are met in the most cost effective way without sacrificing quality.

The Health of the Nation published in 1992 has for the first time set priorities and targets for tackling Britain's major health problems. It will also have an impact on primary health care and therefore on the work of the facilitator.

The Health of the Nation

Published in July 1992 after a six-month consultation period, this white paper puts forward a strategy for improving the general health of the population in England. The document identifies priorities, sets objectives and targets for health, encourages collaboration between organisations, agencies and individuals to implement the strategy and sets out a framework for monitoring and review.

Five key areas have been chosen for action – CHD, cancer, mental illness, HIV/AIDS and sexual health, and accidents. Although other health related problems were considered they did not at the present time meet the criteria of:

- Major causes of premature death or avoidable ill health.
- Amenable to effective intervention.
- Possible to set objectives and targets to monitor progress.

To achieve the targets set, collaboration between statutory and non-statutory organisations is expected in order to maximise the impact on the nation's health. DHAs and FHSAs under the guidance of RHAs are expected to:

- Develop and agree local health service targets.
- Develop purchasing and health investment plans.
- Ensure the focus of health care provision is shifted towards health promotion.

RHAs are expected to assist the process of collaboration where necessary, provide support to the profession and promote research and development.

THE TARGETS

Coronary heart disease and stroke (Baseline 1990)

By the year 2000 to reduce mortality from:

- CHD and stroke in people under 65 by 40 per cent.
- CHD in people aged 65–74 by 30 per cent.
- Stroke in people aged 65–74 by 40 per cent.

Cancers

By the year 2000 to reduce:

- Mortality from breast cancer in the population invited for screening, by 25 per cent. (Baseline 1990.)

- The incidence of invasive cervical cancer by 20 per cent. (Baseline 1986.)
- Mortality from lung cancer by 30 per cent in men and 15 per cent in women aged under 75 years. (Baseline 1990.)
- To halt year on year increse in the incidence of skin cancer by the year 2005.

Mental illness
(Baseline 1990)

- To improve the health and social functioning of mentally ill people.
- To reduce the overall suicide rate by 15 per cent by the year 2000.
- To reduce the suicide rate of severely mentally ill people by 33 per cent by the year 2000.

HIV/AIDS and sexual health

To reduce:
- The incidence of gonorrhoea by 20 per cent by 1995 as an indicator of HIV/AIDS trends. (Baseline 1990.)
- Pregnancy by 50 per cent in the under 16 age group by the year 2000. (Baseline 1989.)

Accidents
(Baseline 1990)

By the year 2005, to reduce mortality from accidents in:

- Children under 15 by 33 per cent.
- The 15–24 age group by 25 per cent.
- The population over 65 by 33 per cent.

Risk factors

Targets have also been set for:

- Smoking.
- Diet and nutrition.
- Blood pressure.
- HIV/AIDS.

RESOURCES

There are several aimed at helping primary care managers and primary health care teams to address the issues identified in *The Health of the Nation.*

Better Living, Better Life (Field & Henderson, 1993) is the main resource available for primary health care teams. This is a useful publication in a number of ways as it gives a great deal of background information on the major causes of mortality and morbidity as well as practical steps to take in addressing these areas. Each practice should have one. Copies are available from your FHSA.

Also the DOH has issued handbooks covering the five key target areas. These are available from HMSO and other good bookshops and are intended to assist managers and directors in purchasing authorities to develop local strategies for these areas.

The role of the FHSA

As part of the NHS review, in September 1990 the FPC became known as the FHSA, of which there are 98 in England and Wales. The Scottish system is different in that the functions of DHA and FHSA are combined and known as a Health Board. Usually the administrative areas of FHSAs are co-terminous with county boundaries or metropolitan district boundaries.

Of the 90 FHSAs in England, 60 relate to one or two DHAs; 17 relate to seven DHAs; three to four DHAs and six relate to five or more DHAs. This situation is likely to change however as FHSAs and DHAs merge their purchasing function, or become one authority following proposed legislation in 1994.

FAMILY PRACTITIONER SERVICES

The limited role of the FPC included the statutory responsibility to administer arrangements for providing general medical, dental, ophthalmic and pharmaceutical services. Their main duties consisted of:

- Maintaining lists of practitioners.
- Providing information to the public.
- Paying practitioners and ensuring compliance with their contracts.
- Dealing with complaints made by patients.
- Maintaining details of patients registered with GPs and arranging the transfer of patients' records.

Membership

The committee usually comprised of 30 people – half professional and half lay-members. The chairperson was appointed separately by the Secretary of State. The FPC was responsible directly to the DOH.

FHSAs

GPs continue to be independent contractors and not employees of the NHS, but the terms and conditions under which they work are negotiated nationally and FHSAs are responsible for implementing the national contracts in their area.

Under the NHS reforms the role of FHSAs has been strengthened in various ways. They have responsibility for:

- Authorising and monitoring the use of deputising services.
- Ensuring the standards of premises are maintained.
- Approving surgery locations and hours of availability.
- Controlling and managing funds for practice developments, including practice staff and premises.

The development of primary health care services is seen as an increasingly important role for the NHS.

Assessing health needs of the population

Working for Patients highlights the responsibility of FHSAs to ensure community involvement in the continuing identification of health problems and priorities. Part of this process should involve developing methods of increasing knowledge and awareness of services provided and to ensure these services are accessible by the population. In this way 'consumers' should be able to exercise choice of a wide range of services to best suit their needs. One of their prime tasks in the coming years will be to work with DHAs to ensure that the health needs of the population they serve are assessed and that services are developed to meet those needs.

Quality commitment

FHSAs are required to ensure that quality indicators are integrated into all primary health care programmes. They have a much strengthened planning and management role to ensure delivery of efficient and effective services and should monitor the standard of those services ensuring greater collaboration between HAs, service providers and consumer groups.

Management of GP fundholding

Since 1991, one of the most important functions of the FHSA has been to work with the RHA on the introduction of fundholding practices. Practices with over 9000 patients who are eligible for fundholding, are able to purchase hospital services for their patients and manage their own practice budget. The FHSAs role has been to assist RHAs in managing this process. It should be noted however that fundholding remains entirely voluntary.

Health promotion

Promoting Better Health and *Working for Patients* emphasise the role of FHSAs in encouraging health promotion activities in primary care. *The Health of the Nation* and the supporting key target area documents, have provided the strategic direction for the focus of preventive activity and health promotion work. Some FHSAs have set up their own health promotion unit. Primary care facilitators may work within this unit or as part of the service development team. There is generally a professional accountability to the nurse or medical adviser director.

Government policies have increasingly focused on health promotion and disease prevention. The FHSA has for a number of years been responsible for the administration of screening programmes for cervical cancer and most are now involved in co-ordinating the call and recall of women for breast cancer screening.

GPs have been encouraged, with financial incentives, to give priorities to health promotion. Primary care facilitators usually take on a supportive role within general practice in order to develop these services.

The FHSA will take a key role in monitoring the new health promotion banding arrangements, which were introduced in July 1993. The banding will be discussed in the following section.

Membership

The membership of the FHSA has been changed to reflect their new role. The authority now comprises only five lay non-executive members, and four professional non-executive members (a GP, dentist, pharmacist and community nurse) appointed by the RHA. The chairman continues to be appointed by the Secretary of State.

Management structure

This likewise reflects the enhanced role and responsibility of the FHSA. The senior officer is the General Manager or Chief Executive. FHSAs have appointed directors with responsibility for developing specific areas of activity, for example, a Director of Finance, Director of Service Development and Planning, Information and Planning, or Director of Administration. There

DOH

Policy and advice to authorities.
Allocation of resources.
Monitoring performance of authorities.

RHAs

Planning the development of services
and implementing national guide-lines.
Allocating resources of DHA, FHSA and
GP Fundholders.
Monitoring performance of DHA and
FHSA.
Research and development.

DHA

Purchasing services for the district
population.
Managing units which remain directly
under their control.
Assessing health needs.
Public Health.

FHSAs

Managing GP contracts.
Assessing health needs.
Planning services to meet health needs.
Managing GP development funds.

NHS Trust

Preparation of business plans.
Submission of annual reports and
accounts.
Improvement of the quality of services
provided to patients.

Special H A s

Functions differ according to specifiic
area of activity.
All responsible directly to Secretary of
State.

Established to represent public interest in
local premises of health services.
Little formal power but seek to influence
decision of DHAs and FHSAs through
advice and information.

CHCs

* Major restructuring of the HAs was announced towards the end of 1993. The number of RHAs will reduce from 14 to eight, and DHAs and FHSAs can merge once the Act of Parliament has been passed in 1994.

Figure 1.1. Summary of functions of health department and HAs in England*

may also be a Consumer Affairs Manager, Operational Manager, a Quality Assurance Manager and a number of advisers usually drawn from the professions, for example, medical adviser, pharmacy adviser, nurse adviser.

SUMMARY

A summary of the organisation of the NHS in England is given in Fig. 1.1 (adapted from Ham, 1991).

The GP contract

New contractual arrangements for GPs, introduced on 1st April 1990, are beginning to change the relationship between individual GPs, the FHSA and the public. Emphasis has been placed on the provision of 'consumer' (patient) information, accountability and the range of services GPs are required to provide for their patients. The following summary is intended to provide information which may be useful to you in your work. It describes the range of services GPs provide under the 1990 contract and some of the arrangements whereby GPs can claim reimbursement for developing additional services. It is not intended to be a full account of GP payment arrangements as this is unlikely to be relevant to you in your role as facilitator. It is advisable, whether or not you are employed by an FHSA to enquire about local arrangements which may differ from what has been detailed here. Full details of fees and allowances can be found in the *Statement of Fees and Allowances (Department of Health, 1990b)* otherwise known as the 'Red Book'.

SUMMARY OF THE CONTRACT AND ITS IMPLICATIONS

Consumer information

Practice leaflets
GPs are required to produce a practice leaflet which should be reviewed annually to maintain accuracy. The leaflet should normally include information about the services provided by the GP and/or the primary health care team, including surgery times, times of specific clinics and the availability of other team members. The leaflets must be made available to every patient on the doctor's list and the general public via the FHSA.

Local directories
Information is provided by the GP for inclusion in a directory of general medical practitioners. These directories are then made available to the public at the FHSA, in local libraries and health establishments.

Accountability

Annual reports
A GP is required to provide the FHSA with an annual report containing information about:

- The practice staff including number, duties and qualifications.
- The practice premises.
- The activity of the practice, particularly in relation to referral patterns.
- Commitments other than within the practice by the doctor – e.g., posts held elsewhere.
- How the doctor receives comments from the patients, on the services offered.
- Information in respect of prescribing of drugs and appliances.

Medical audit
This remains outside the contractual obligations of the GP at present.

MAAGs appointed by FHSAs are charged with the task of 'encouraging' all practices to undertake medical audit. Although medical audit has been portrayed as an educational activity there are concerns among the medical profession that audit is one way to seek out 'bad apples'. The profession argues however that monitoring standards should be the profession's own responsibility.

Indicative drug prescribing
A doctor is free within reason to prescribe any drug he deems necessary to the care of his patient with the exception of those which appear on a 'forbidden list', that is, schedule 3A to the regulations. GPs are, however, sent detailed breakdowns of their prescribing activity by the prescription pricing authority (PACT data), which can be compared to the district and national average. The medical advisor is responsible for ensuring doctors are prescribing appropriately, and are able to stay within an indicative prescribing amount, based on previous years' spending.

Other aspects of accountability

- On receiving a written request from the FHSA, GPs must allow the premises to be visited at any reasonable time by a representative of the FHSA or LMC or both.
- Practitioners must notify the FHSA of any proposed changes in service arrangements, for example, significant changes in appointment systems or proposals to discontinue certain systems.
- Random visits can be made to patients to verify claims for out-of-hours visits.

Services to patients

Availability
GPs must be available to their patients for 42 weeks in any twelve months, and for not less than 26 hours over five days of the week. The hours of availability must also be at times convenient to their patients and in any case, must be approved by the FHSA.

Type of service provided
GPs are required to provide their patients with all necessary personal medical services and are responsible for the care of their patients 24 hours a day.

They have a duty to arrange an 'on call' service to patients when not personally available. They are normally expected to treat patients within the defined practice area which includes home visits.

There is no obligation for GPs to provide contraceptive services, child health surveillance, minor surgery or maternity services or specific health promotion clinics unless they have previously agreed to do so. The GP is now required, however, *to offer* (by way of a written invitation) to:

- *Newly registered patients* (over 5 years of age), within 28 days of registration with the doctor, a consultation to,
  – obtain details of past medical history, social factors and lifestyle factors which may affect health;
  – assess the patient's current health status by physical examination including height, weight, blood pressure and urinalysis;
  – record the findings within the patient's notes;
  – offer to discuss the conclusions of the consultation with the patient and to assess the need for personal medical services.
- *Patients not seen within 3 years* (aged between 16–75) a similar consultation to the one listed above. (*This aspect of the GP contract has now been scrapped.*)

● *Patients aged 75 years and over* (within 12 months of their 75th birthday or 12 months of joining the GPs list if already over 75).

The GP should offer, in writing, a consultation and domiciliary visit (which may be combined) to assess factors affecting the patient's general health including:

● sensory functions;
● mobility;
● mental condition;
● physical condition;
● social environment;
● use of medicines.

Also the GP should record the findings and offer to discuss with the patient conclusions drawn from the consultation.

Some of these new services, for example three-yearly checks, have however been opposed by many in primary care, as it has been argued that they have no scientific validity to support them. The contract is under discussion at present and it is expected that some of these contractual obligations will be withdrawn.

Non-contractual services to patients

Usually these services attract specific fees over and above the basic practice allowance and capitation fees. The services offered are as follows.

Maternity medical services
A GP must seek admission to the obstetric list in order to provide maternity medical services to patients; this requires having the GP's experience in obstetrics approved by the local obstetric committee or the Secretary of State for Health.

Contraceptive services

Child health surveillance
A doctor wishing to provide child health surveillance for children up to five years of age and be paid for such services, must apply to be included on the FHSA's child health surveillance list. A separate list of such patients is maintained by the FHSA. The GP must agree to:

● Provide a monitoring service while the child is below five years of age with the view to detecting any deviations from normal development. This surveillance may be carried out by an appropriately qualified person on the doctor's behalf.

- Keep accurate records of the examinations carried out.

- Provide the health authority with a survey of the procedures and findings of each examination.

Minor surgery

A doctor must be included in FHSA's minor surgery list in order to claim a fee for performing minor surgical procedures.

No more than three sessions can be claimed in any quarter. A session consists of five surgical procedures from a specified list which includes certain injections, aspirations, incisions, excisions, curette, cautery and cryocautery.

Health promotion

Advice on lifestyle and general health education should be provided, where appropriate, opportunistically by GPs within the normal consultation. The new contract introduced a separate fee which was payable to GPs for each health promotion clinic they or a suitably qualified member of their staff provided. Health promotion in this context refers to surveillance, detection of risk factors for disease, general advice and counselling on the maintenance of good health, chronic disease management and tertiary prevention.

Some services which are separately remunerated do not qualify for this payment, for example, maternity medical services and cervical cytology. There has been considerable debate about the quality and appropriateness of such clinics and FHSAs interpreted the Department's recommendations in a number of different ways. These arrangements, however, have had their difficulties, with no easy way to monitor their appropriateness or effectiveness.

From 1st July 1993, a new system came into operation, whereby GPs are paid according to a specific practice strategy in order to improve recording of certain risk factors and develop services which are appropriate to their own population needs. This is discussed in detail in the next section.

Cervical cytology

Individual cytology tests are no longer eligible for payment under the new contract arrangements. Instead, payment is calculated according to a system of targets for level of uptake. The higher rate is payable if 80 per cent of eligible (i.e. aged between 25 and 64) women on the GP's list have had an 'adequate' smear during the preceding 5.5 years. A lower payment is made if at least 50 per cent of eligible women have had an adequate test. (Excluded from the calculation of eligible women, are those who have had hyster-ectomies involving removal of cervix.)

Immunisation for children aged two and under
A target payment is also in operation for this category. A GP will receive payment at the higher rate if the number of courses completed in specified groups of immunisation is on average 90 per cent of those children who are eligible. The lower payment is given if only 70 per cent are immunised.

Pre-school boosters for children aged five and under
Similar target payments are payable for the pre-school boosters.

Although many GPs have responded well to their target system, those working in inner city areas have particular difficulties in achieving them.

POSTGRADUATE EDUCATION ALLOWANCE

In order to encourage GPs to continue postgraduate education, the 1990 Contract introduced the PGEA. GPs are eligible for the allowance after attending 25 days 'accredited' postgraduate education, spread over a period of five years. During that time the GP has to attend at least two courses in each of the following categories:

- Health promotion and the prevention of illness.
- Disease management.
- Service management.

If the GP does not satisfy the full criteria for the allowance he or she will still be eligible for an apportioned amount.

Courses which qualify for PGEA approval

Courses are approved by the Regional Advisor for Postgraduate Education, or in Wales the Postgraduate Dean. Applications are sent to the Advisor, who decides whether the course meets the criteria for approval, the number of days accreditation it should be awarded and the categories into which the session falls.

The service management section includes, for example, record systems, use of technology, staff management, practice organisation, quality assurance and audit. As it is often difficult for GPs to attend courses which take them away from their normal surgery commitments, approval has been given for a variety of formats. These range from conferences or courses with straight lectures and for group work to more informal sessions held in the GP surgery. Sometimes accreditation is given to a series of meetings or study sessions each of a short duration but held over longer periods of time. A full day's accreditation consists of six hours excluding tea breaks and lunch.

Most regions request substantial notice for PGEA approval of a course or seminar. As a facilitator you are advised to contact the postgraduate dean early in the planning stages of your training event. Before approval can be given you will be expected to submit a detailed plan of the course including the learning objectives, content and duration of each session.

There is some variation, however, between regions about the exact criteria for PGEA approval. You will need to contact your postgraduate dean or regional adviser to find out exactly how it works in your area.

If approval is given it will be your responsibility to ensure that GPs sign the attendance register and they are issued with a certificate of attendance. The register, together with course evaluations are then sent back to the Regional Postgraduate Dean.

PRACTICE STAFF

Under the new practice staff scheme the FHSA can, at their discretion, reimburse all or part of the expenses incurred by GPs employing practice staff (other than those undertaking medical duties). This can include salary, National Insurance and NHS superannuation contributions, staff training, holiday pay, sick pay and maternity benefit. However, the practice staff budget is now a cash limited resource and FHSAs are required to ensure resources are targeted to address the health needs of patients.

Under the new scheme, FHSAs can reimburse the costs of employing a wider range of staff, including for example, physiotherapists, chiropodists, dietitians, counsellors, translators.

COMPUTERS

A proportion of the costs incurred by general practitioners to buy, lease, upgrade or maintain a computer system or to employ staff to set up the system, can be reimbursed on a scale according to list size. It is not usually more than 50 per cent.

Health promotion banding arrangements

New health promotion arrangements have come into effect from 1st July 1993. The aim has been to:

- Set GP health promotion activity within a strategic framework reflecting *The Health of the Nation* priorities.
- Offer greater freedom for different health promotion approaches and to ensure effective targeting of resources.
- Promote equality of access.
- Ensure allocation of resources is predictable.

Remuneration depends on the 'Band' the practice achieves.

HEALTH PROMOTION ACTIVITY

- Band 1, is concerned with providing smoking reduction programmes.
- Band 2, is aimed at reducing morbidity and mortality from hypertension and established CHD or stroke.
- Band 3, is concerned with developing a comprehensive CHD and stroke prevention strategy.

Each of the bands includes the collection of 'relevant' information on 15 to 74-year-olds, encourages working with other individuals or agencies to achieve the practice goals, and should focus on priority groups and patients who do not attend the surgeries.

CHRONIC DISEASE MANAGEMENT

There is also a fixed payment per GP for organised diabetes and asthma care within the practice.

GENERAL POINTS

Single practices may join with other practices to offer joint programmes. There will be a cash limit on payment for health promotion, and payment is apportioned according to list size. Limited transitional payments are available during the first year to compensate those GPs whose earnings presently exceed the new limits. Each practice must apply annually for inclusion in the appropriate band. Evaluation of the work is implicit and practices must audit their programme and provide the FHSA with aggregate data.

Banding proposals are subject to local interpretation; further information is available from your local FHSA.

2 The nature of disease and health promotion

Epidemiology

WHAT IS EPIDEMIOLOGY?

The word epidemiology is derived from Greek and means literally 'studies upon people'. In contrast to clinical medicine, it involves the study of groups of people (populations) rather than the direct study of individuals.

While clinical observations provide information about individuals and their response to disease, epidemiological observations aim to answer questions about why a disease affects one person rather than another, why it occurs in one country rather than another or why in winter rather than summer. Epidemiologists monitor trends in disease patterns to show whether diseases are increasing or decreasing in frequency and to monitor changes in distribution. Two important concepts are involved in epidemiological research – cause and risk.

Cause of disease

In order to distinguish an association between causal factors and disease, the following factors need to be examined.

- Time sequence – the time taken for exposure to a causal agent, to the onset of disease.
- Distribution – the distribution of the disease and its correlation with the amount and duration of exposure, with the suspected causal agent.
- Consistency – the association found between a causal agent and disease occurring in different populations.
- Plausibility – the association between the disease and the suspected causal agent and its consistency with the known activity of that agent.
- Preventive trials – the decreasing incidence of disease, resulting from the removal or control of the suspected agent.

Risk

There are three common indices of risk:

- Absolute risk
  This is the incidence rate of the disease among people exposed to the causal agent. It assumes, however, that no risk is incurred by people not exposed to the risk.

- Relative risk
  This is an estimate of the magnitude of an association between exposure and disease. In other words, how likely it is that a person will contract the disease having been exposed to the disease, or causes of a disease, relative to someone who has not been exposed. This is the ratio of the incidence of disease in an exposed group divided by the incidence in the non-exposed group.

- Attributable risk
  This is the absolute effect of exposure in the exposed group compared with those not exposed. In other words, the incidence of disease in the exposed group less the incidence of disease in the non-exposed group.

METHODS OF DESCRIPTION

The *prevalence rate* is the proportion of people in a population who are affected by a disease *at one point in time* (point prevalence) or *over a period of time* (period prevalence).

The *incidence rate* is the proportion of the population developing a condition *within a stated period* and it measures *the rate of occurrence of new cases*.

MEASURING DISEASE

The rate consists of three components:

- A numerator – the number of people in the population who experience events concerned with, for example, deaths, cases of disease or births.
- A denominator – the total number of people in the population being considered.
- The time period – during which the events took place.

So that:

$$\frac{\text{Number of deaths (numerator) in the year (time period)}}{\text{Number of people in the total population (denominator)}} = \begin{array}{l}\text{The annual} \\ crude \text{ death} \\ \text{rate}\end{array}$$

CRUDE RATES

'Crude' here implies that the rate concerns the entire population of the geographical area being considered. This figure is usually multiplied by 1000 and expressed as an amount per thousand population.

What this measurement does not provide, however, is anything about the characteristics of the population which may affect this rate, as for example, the proportion of elderly in the population. Caution is therefore needed when making comparisons between populations.

SPECIFIC RATES

A specific rate refers to the number of events occurring in a subgroup of the population. Age and sex linked to cause are the most commonly described subgroup, but occupation, social class and race are also used. Likewise death rates may be expressed for individual causes of death rather than all cause rates.

Comparisons are frequently made between populations using age, sex and specific cause.

STANDARDISED RATES

These take account of the age structures of a population, so that their mortality experience can be compared directly with another similar population. By using a suitable reference population the number of 'observed' deaths is compared to the number of 'expected' deaths. The ratio between the two figures, expressed as a percentage, is called the SMR.

Values over 100 per cent represent unfavourable mortality and values below 100 per cent represent favourable mortality risk. (The effects of age and usually sex have been taken into account.) A worked example is provided in Table 2.1.

TYPES OF EPIDEMIOLOGICAL STUDY

● Retrospective studies – measure what happened in the past and draw conclusions from data already available.

● Case controlled studies – use two groups, where one group has the condition being studied and the other group has not. The two groups, however, must be matched on all other counts which may otherwise affect the conclusions which can be drawn.

Table 2.1 Calculation of SMR for two occupational groups

(A) Original data 1959–63

Occupation	Number in occupational group (from census)	Observed deaths	Crude death rate/1000 per annum
Farmers, Foresters and Fishermen	705,910	20,973	5.9
Armed Forces	301,120	4,282	2.8

This suggests a lower mortality in the armed forces.

(B) Calculation of expected number of deaths

Age (years)	Farmers, foresters, fishermen			Armed forces	
	Annual death rates/1000 in men (England and Wales) (from national mortality statistics)	Number in occupation group	Number of expected deaths* in occupation 1959–63	Number in occupation group	Number of expected deaths* in occupation 1959–63
15–24	1,028	134,560	691.6	165,030	848.3
25–34	1,118	124,100	693.7	73,240	409.4
35–44	2,411	132,220	1,593.9	42,250	509.3
45–54	7,072	150,110	5,661.5	15,930	563.3
55–64	21,710	154,920	16,816.6	4,670	506.9
Total expected deaths			25,457.3		2837.2

*As an *annual* death rate is being used and expected deaths are required for a five-year period (1959–63):

$$\text{Expected deaths} = \frac{\text{Annual death rate in England and Wales} \times \text{Number in age specific group} \times 5}{1000}$$

(C) Calculation of SMR

$$\text{SMR} = \frac{\text{Observed deaths}}{\text{Expected deaths}} \times 100$$

$$\text{SMR Farmers, Foresters, Fishermen} = \frac{20,973}{25457.3} \times 100 = 82$$

$$\text{SMR Armed Forces} = \frac{4282}{2837.2} \times 100 = 151$$

(Cont. p. 23)

- Prospective studies – are used to investigate the *cause* of diseases and are set up to collect information in the future. These studies are normally very accurate because *all* the relevant data can be collected and for long periods of time.

- Intervention studies – are studies where some action is taken and the effects of that action are measured. This is the type of study used in drug trials. Sequential analysis allows the study to be stopped as soon as something is proven.

As individuals can affect the results because of what they 'expect' to happen, 'double blind' trials are sometimes used. This is where for example, one group of people receive a placebo and the other group the drug on trial, but neither the doctor supplying the drug nor the patient knows which one they are to receive. Obviously the ethical considerations have meant that consent is required from those taking part in the trial.

Patterns of disease

Patterns or the distribution of disease are usually described in relation to time, place and person.

TIME

Three common methods are used in epidemiology to examine this relationship.

Long-term trends

Care must be taken when interpreting secular trends in frequency of disease, that is, those newly observed or observed only once. It could be that the frequency of the disease has not changed over time but improvements in methods of detection and diagnosis, for example, suggest it has.

There appears to have been an increase in 'chronic disease', CHD and lung cancer. It may be, however, that this actually reflects an increased awareness of the disease and, in the past, deaths from these sources were attributed to something else.

An important long-term change within industrialised countries during the last century was the decline in deaths from infectious disease.

Table 2.1 (cont.)

There are fewer men in the older age groups in the armed forces, therefore, by adjusting for age (i.e. calculating SMR) there is lower mortality among farmers, foresters and fishermen.

The decline in mortality from TB, however, had begun before specific medical measures were developed to treat and prevent the disease. One must not automatically assume, then, that a decline in the frequency of disease is necessarily due to a specific intervention.

Seasonal variation

Many infectious or communicable diseases vary in occurrence depending on the season. For example, respiratory infections peak in frequency during the colder months.

Some diseases, however, show an apparent seasonal variation but a causal link between an infectious agent and the disease is unclear. The onset of insulin dependent diabetes mellitus, for example, occurs more frequently in the winter months. It may be that the onset of the disease is not precipitated by the season but by an infectious agent, for example, a virus which is more plentiful during that time.

Days or weeks

The sudden increase in the occurrence of a disease that spreads rapidly through a population is referred to as an 'epidemic'. It is usually applied to communicable disease but is sometimes used to describe a disease which is widespread, such as CHD.

PLACE

Patterns of disease are studied in relation to their geography and comparisons are made between them, as follows.

International variation

Disease can vary in occurrence between countries and this often gives clues about causation. It is worth considering, however, how the information from different countries is collected or what methods are used to detect disease, in order to be sure differences are actually due to geographical variations.

National variations

In Britain it has been found that the morbidity and mortality from various diseases vary according to geographical area. For example, chronic bronchitis and CHD are more common in urban, industrial areas of northern England than in the rural south of England. In general, mortality within Britain is higher in the North and northwest of England, Wales and Scotland than in the South and East Anglia. The reason is multifactoral and, as such, very complex.

Lower social class, poor housing, high levels of unemployment and poor nutrition in those areas appear to contribute significantly to the high levels of morbidity.

Variations in mortality between areas are simply expressed using SMR.

Local (urban/rural) variations

District-wide figures are held by the Department of Public Health Medicine who in some areas also produce variations in patterns of disease within small areas, that is, the urban and rural population of their districts or between electoral wards.

Recent NHS changes have made this type of analysis the responsibility of the Department of Public Health Medicine. Morbidity data will form an essential part of health needs assessment along with population surveys and information on referral patterns from hospital or general practice.

PERSON

Most diseases show a distinct variation in frequency according to age, sex, occupation and social class. Some diseases vary according to marital status, and among individuals of different ethnic origin. Examples include:

- Age – chronic degenerative diseases; disease of the circulation, cancer and respiratory disease (more common in advancing years); accidents; deaths due to violence; certain cancers that are more common in younger age groups.

- Sex – despite the decline in mortality in both sexes for all ages over time, the ratio of male to female mortality has been increasing. In particular, deaths from road accidents are more common in young adult males and from CHD and lung cancer in middle to later years. Cultural and behavioural factors such as cigarette smoking and use of motor vehicles may be the reason for maintaining the difference.

- Occupation and social class – occupation has been used as a means of determining social class in Britain since the beginning of the twentieth century and is collected by census, registration of births and deaths. The information relates to the persons present or most recent occupation. From this information, health can be studied according to the direct hazards of different occupations or in relation to lifestyle factors normally associated with different social groups.

The major causes of death and morbidity in this country are diseases of the circulation, including CHD and strokes, and cancer, including cancer of the lung, breast and stomach.

CHD

Is responsible for one in three deaths among men and one in four deaths among women, which represents 27 per cent of all deaths (Coronary Prevention Group, 1990) in the UK. It remains the main cause of premature death in the UK for men (1 in 12 before the age of 65) and, after cancer, is the leading cause of premature death among women (1 in 45 women before the age of 65).

Mortality from CHD in the UK is among the highest in the world. Since 1968, the USA and Australia, both previously with higher rates of mortality from CHD than the UK, have reduced the death rates by half among the 35–74 age group. Death rates in other countries, for example, New Zealand, Japan and Finland are also falling at a rate substantially greater than those in the UK. Deaths due to CHD in the UK, by comparison, have fallen by only 12 per cent in England and Wales, 9 per cent in Scotland and 7 per cent in Northern Ireland.

CHD was responsible for about 26 per cent of deaths in England in 1991, accounting for 2.5 per cent of the total NHS expenditure and has resulted in 35 million lost working days each year. Strokes accounted for 12 per cent of all deaths in 1991, which is also a major cause of disability, especially among the elderly. Patterns of CHD varies within the UK according to region, social class, ethnic origin and age.

Causes

The identification of factors which cause or are closely and consistently associated with CHD, has been the aim of numerous research studies. Before any factor can be described as truly causal it must satisfy a number of stringent criteria. In CHD a number of factors have been found to be associated with an increased presence or emergence of the disease. These are known as risk factors. Not all risk factors have the same strength of relationship with CHD or can be shown to be truly causal. It has become widely accepted that CHD is a 'multi-factorial disease'. That is, there are many factors associated with increased prevalence of the disease, some of which may interact with one another to increase the likelihood of developing the disease. The main risk factors associated with CHD and stroke are:

- Age
- Race } not modifiable
- Sex

- Smoking
- Blood cholesterol
- High blood pressure } modifiable
- Obesity
- Lack of exercise

Other risk factors, such as socio-economic factors, influence from early life and stress are less well understood. The Black report, however, proved that higher levels of ill health are to be found in areas of social deprivation (Townsend & Davidson, 1982).

Cigarette smoking and CHD

Research studies relating to causes of CHD have shown that:

- Smoking is an independent risk factor for CHD and may act as a synergist with high blood pressure and raised cholesterol.
- Cigarette smoking increases atheroma formation in the coronary arteries.
- Smoking is dose-related in its contribution towards risk of acute MI.
- Smokers are at greater risk (compared to non-smokers) of developing angina pectoris.

Hypertension

Raised systolic and diastolic blood pressures increase the risk of CHD and stroke in both sexes. In the British Regional Heart Study (Shaper *et al.*, 1982), CHD risk was increased two-fold with a systolic blood pressure of over 148 mmHg or with a diastolic blood pressure of over 93 mmHg.

Serum cholesterol

High concentrations of serum cholesterol increase the risk of death from CHD. More than 70 per cent of the population of the UK have levels of serum cholesterol greater than 5.2 mmols/litre. Serum cholesterol lower than 5.2 mmols/litre still carry some risk, but this level has become the accepted target in Western communities. A more sensitive indicator of risk can be derived from measuring

HDL and LDL. Increased levels of LDL fractions of cholesterol increase coronary risk while increased levels of HDL reduces it. The relatively uncommon inherited condition, familial hyperlipidemia, affects 1 in 500 people.

The link between raised serum cholesterol and the intake of dietary fat is complex. In Western countries, the evidence suggests that where the diet is high in saturated (mainly animal) fats rather than polyunsaturated (mainly vegetable) fats (i.e. with a low polyunsaturated:saturated fat ratio), CHD is high. Conversely, populations with low saturated fat intake and a high polyunsaturated to saturated fat ratio, show a low incidence of CHD.

The role of dietary cholesterol and its effect on CHD risk in individuals is more difficult to assess. There is considerable variation between individuals in their ability to absorb and metabolise cholesterol. There is, however, sufficient epidemiological evidence, to suggest that atherosclerosis primarily related to nutrition is to some extent avoidable and can be halted using dietary measures. Evidence from clinical trials has not been conclusive, however, and the debate therefore continues.

A systematic review and synthesis of literature relating to cholesterol screening and treatment has been published by the University of Leeds for the Department of Health in the *Effective Health Care* bulletin (Sheldon *et al.*, 1993). It makes the following points:

- Blood cholesterol is an important risk factor for CHD but should be considered in the context of other risk factors such as smoking, raised blood pressure and inactivity. By itself it is a poor predictor of individual risk of CHD.

- Cholesterol screening programmes have been introduced without sufficient evaluation and few people identified purely on the basis of cholesterol levels, will benefit from treatment.

- Cholesterol screening will not make a contribution to the lowering of overall mortality and should be actively discouraged.

Obesity

Risk of CHD increases in individuals who are above 'average' weight for height. Nevertheless, this may be largely to do with the likelihood of associated high blood pressure, raised serum cholesterol and lack of physical activity. Evidence that obesity is an independent risk factor is poor, but remains an important risk indicator.

Exercise

There is considerable evidence to suggest that sustained regular physical activity appears to protect against CHD. The exact amount and intensity however remain the subject of debate.

Diabetes

This condition increases the risk of all aspects of CHD although it appears to aggravate the condition rather than act as a causal factor.

Other risk factors

Stress, personality type, water softness, consumption of coffee and alcohol are also claimed to be associated with CHD. There are, however, a variety of conflicting views about their importance.

Better Living, Better Life (Field & Henderson, 1993) and *The Health of the Nation* (DOH, 1992b) provide additional background information particularly relating to the UK, about CHD and risk factors. Resource packs for teaching purposes and patient education literature on alcohol, smoking, exercise and diet is available from the HEA and can be requested directly from them (see Chapter 7).

SUMMARY

Summaries of CHD research trials and their approaches to prevention are presented in Tables 2.2, 2.3 and 2.4.

All the trials aimed at reducing the incidence of CHD have had limited success. This could be due to the method of selection for the trials or that they have mostly focused on high risk as defined by levels of serum TC or cholesterol and smoking, rather than in a multi-factorial way. All the trials, however, show that changes in personal behaviour or lifestyle can lead to a reduction in the incidence of CHD.

Combined with epidemiological evidence and clinical evidence from work with individuals, this is probably sufficient to prompt action in order to attempt to prevent CHD.

Sources of health information

There is no single source that provides a full range of health information. This is hardly surprising. Few information systems have been designed to provide detailed information about the health needs or problems of a population, however, the recent

Table 2.2 The early studies – CHD research trials using unifactoral interventions

Trial	Year	Design	Result
Los Angeles Veterans Administration Study	1969	Random, control, double blind trial, 846 men ages 54–88 years. Experimental group given diet with p/s ratio* 2:1. *Duration*: 8 years	Beneficial effect of cholesterol lowering diet on under 65s who had higher serum cholesterol levels at the start of the study. Significantly more deaths and non-fatal events had occurred in the control group.
Finnish Mental Hospitals Study	1979	700 men and 600 women (aged 34–64) drawn from two Helsinki Mental hospitals. Experimental group given dietary information and p/s ratio 2:1 diet for 6 years. Then repeated on control groups for further 6 years. *Duration*: 12 years	Moderately beneficial effect on CHD and stroke in men on experimental diet with a small effect on women. However, other variables – changes in patient composition in the hospitals – led to problems associated with analysis of the data.

*p/s ratio = polyunsaturated to saturated fat ratio

NHS reforms have established this as a priority aim. Little of the information that has been collected has been available to build a full picture on which to plan health care services. Although population, mortality and morbidity data are collected routinely from a number of sources they still have limitations.

POPULATION DATA

The census is the most important source of information on the size and composition of the population. It is co-ordinated by OPCS. Information is available about age, sex, marital status, nationality, occupation and employment status, higher education, means of

Table 2.3 CHD research trials using the unifactorial community approach

Trial	Year	Design	Result
North Karelia Project (Finland)	1972–82 (continuing)	Surveys of representative population and samples (10,000) each time in 1972, 77 and 82. Whole population involvement for community action against CHD risk factors using mass media and environmental services to support lifestyle change. Outcome compared to neighbouring county. *Duration*: 5–10 years, and continuing	Reduction in risk factors was generally greater in North Karelia than Kilopia – particularly cigarette smoking. CHD mortality and incidence of acute MI* and stroke were decreased but not significantly more than control. N. Karelia showed a 22% reduction in age standardised CHD mortality in men compared with 12% in Kilopia and 11% the rest of Finland. The reduction was less marked in women. The subsequent survey in 1982 showed that these effects persisted after 10 years.
WHO European Collaborative Trial	1986	49,781 men aged 40–59 years working in paired factories in UK, Belgium, Italy, Spain and Poland Each pair = one intervention and one control factory. Factories were randomised so that health education could be given to a whole group without risk of influencing control factories. *Duration*: 6 years	There was an average reduction in estimated CHD risk of 11% in the intervention group and for men at high risk the reduction was 22%. There were differences, however, in the success of reducing risk factors between countries. The reduction in both total CHD and total mortality was significant only in Belgium. The results also indicate that different cultures respond differently to advice and lifestyle.

*MI = myocardial infarction

Table 2.4 CHD research trials using the high risk approach

Trial	Year	Design	Result
WHO co-operative trial using clofibrate	1978	Study of primary prevention where serum cholesterol levels were to be lowered by clofibrate. 15,745 healthy men aged 30–59 years from Edinburgh, Budapest and Prague. Assigned to three groups according to their serum TC levels*. Double blind randomised control trial. *Duration*: 5 years.	Significant reduction of major non-fatal CHD in those given clofibrate compared with placebo group but no difference in fatal cases and an *increase* in all causes of mortality. While providing reasonable evidence that lowering lipids reduces incidence of CHD the study threw grave doubts on the use of drugs in primary prevention.
Oslo study	1981	1232 normotensive healthy Norwegian men at high risk of CHD (aged 40–49). Randomized trial to reduce smoking and serum cholesterol. (Men had initial serum cholesterol levels of 7.5–9.8 mmol/L and 80% smoked cigarettes.) *Duration*: 5 years.	TC levels were 13% lower and number of cigarettes smoked/day was 45% lower in the intervention group. There was a 47% reduction in fatal and non-fatal CHD. Reduction in CHD incidence was shown to be due largely to lipid lowering. There was *no statistical* significance in corornary events between the two groups. Some decrease in events was noted.

(Cont'd)

(**Table 2.4** *cont.*)

Trial	Year	Design	Result
Multiple Risk Factor Intervention Trial (MRFIT)	1982	12,866 high risk men (based on smoking, BP* and serum cholesterol concentration) aged 35–57 but with no evidence of CHD. Half the men randomly allocated to intervention group receiving 4-monthly check ups and advice on stopping smoking, controlling BP and altering diet to reduce hyper-cholesterolaemia. The control group were told risk status and may have received advice from own GPs. *7 year* follow up.	Smoking, BP and serum TC were decreased in both groups though significantly more in intervention group. CHD mortality (after 7 years follow up) was reduced by 22% more in intervention group though this was not statistically significant. In retrospect the control group was unsatisfactory thus making it difficult to detect a significant difference between the two.
Lipid Research Clinics Study	1984	3806 American men aged 35–59 with serum TC levels > 6.85 mmol/L were randomised into two groups for a double blind trial. One received cholestyramine, the other control group received a placebo. Both groups followed a cholesterol lowering diet. *Duration*: 7 years	In the drug treated group there was (i) 19% lower incidence of fatal and non-fatal CHD events; (ii) 20% fewer causes of angina; (iii) serum cholesterol levels were 9% lower; (iv) 21% fewer coronary bypass operations. There was no statistical signi-ficance, however, in development of CHD.

*BP = blood pressure; Serum TC levels = serum total cholesterol levels transport to work and housing. This is used to plan such things as housing, schools, pensions and social security, as well as health and social services.

Census data provides information on the whole population. It falls short, however, of 100 per cent coverage. Census forms are sent to households, thereby missing the homeless, and the information provided in some cases is inaccurate, particularly age, marital status and occupation. A further limiting factor is that the census takes place only every 10 years although interim population estimates are produced on a yearly basis using other sources of information concerning mortality, fertility and marriage. The information can be broken down into smaller statistical areas including by RHA, DHA, ward or parish. In the health field, therefore, these statistics can be used for planning health services, for example, hospitals, health centres, numbers of GPs, health visitors and district nurses. The composition of the population provides crude indicators of need for health and social services for quite small geographical areas.

The OPCS publishes this type of information on a regular basis and it is usually available from a health promotion/education unit, Department of Public Health Medicine, the FHSA or the District Health Information Office.

MORTALITY DATA

Mortality refers to the number of *deaths* within a population. Again collection of this data is organised by the OPCS but this time it is collected locally by registrars appointed by each local authority. Following certification by a medical practitioner, a 'qualified informant' (usually a close relative of the deceased) presents the registrar with details of the deceased's name, sex, date and place of birth, occupation and place of residence and the medical certificate stating cause of death, and any other significant conditions which may have contributed to the death. When the cause of death is unknown or the deceased has not seen a doctor during the week prior to the death, it must be reported to the coroner, who may order a post mortem. This information is sent weekly to the OPCS where it is coded according to the International Classification of Diseases and the district medical officer of the health district, where the deceased resided.

For over 100 years now, registration of deaths has been required by law. As such an event as death is highly unlikely to be missed, mortality statistics are generally thought to be accurate. However, some of the other information reported to the registrar can be less reliable. Spouses may be prone to misrepresent such details as occupation, for example, and this is used as an indication of social class. As cause of death is based, in most cases, on clinical opinion some inaccuracies can also occur, especially in older people with chronic illness and multiple pathology.

Mortality statistics, however, remain important as they indicate patterns of disease and associations between subgroups of the population, periods of time and geographical spread. The OPCS mortality statistics are available from HMSO bookshops.

VITAL EVENT DATA

In addition, information is also collected by the registrar on births and abortions.

MORBIDITY DATA

Morbidity refers to the number of non-fatal illnesses or diseases affecting a population. It has the potential to provide the rest of the information needed to direct efficient and effective health services planning.

There are a number of sources, again co-ordinated largely by the OPCS, including hospital data, notifications of infectious disease, notification of congenital malformations, the registration of cancers and abortion statistics. Sources other than those related directly to the health service include the general household survey, school medical records, records of industrial injury and occupational disease and the armed forces. The limitations to this data, however, stem from the general lack of systematic recording that presently exists and the inability to find out about those people within the population who do not seek medical advice, use hospital services or have the type of health problems that are not normally recorded in any easily accessible form.

General practice as a source of morbidity data was used in the National Morbidity Study of General Practice in the 1970s, 1980s and in 1992. Information is gathered on patient consultations within the general practice setting. Diagnoses are classified according to the International Classifications of Diseases and other information about referral patterns are studied.

Unfortunately, until now no system has been established to collect this data from practices in a standardised way, even though the potential of this type of information is enormous. The current restructured NHS and primary care services, however, are now beginning to develop new methods of data collection, in the form of general practice annual reports, referral patterns from fundholding practices, prescribing data and to some extent aggregated information from medical audit in primary care. Lack of any centralised control over data collection means that, as yet, information is not standardised and therefore difficult to use. However, FHSAs, DHAs and GPs are being encouraged to collaborate in order to assess the health needs of their population so that planning and priority can be given to the particular needs of any given community. There are also a number of general practice information projects that aim to establish the collection of reliable and accessible data on selected morbidities and risk factors, for example, the Wycombe Project, Surrey FHSA and the Wakefield and Pontefract Primary Care Health Information Project.

The facilitator, however, should not underestimate the information that can be provided from 'unofficial' sources on the health problems of the area he or she serves. Informal discussion with the primary health care team including health visitors, district nurses, practice staff and voluntary agencies working within the area, will highlight areas of need and where services should be developed. Also, the local health promotion unit will be only too pleased to provide information about local health issues.

Health needs assessment

Improving the health of the population includes providing the right services that are accessible to those in need of the service at the most appropriate time. Allocating resources and planning appropriate services has in the past been based on limited information obtained from studying historical patterns of disease and the use of services. The current NHS reforms and particularly the quest for economy and efficiency, have placed much greater emphasis on ensuring health services meet the needs of the population.

HAs are required to review regularly the health of their population in order to make 'rational' decisions about the distribution of resources. This in practice means that contracts will be set on the basis of health needs assessment. The results of those decisions must then be monitored to ensure services provided are meeting the needs of the population and to measure the outcome or 'health gain' (i.e. the achievement of a measurable improvement in the health of the population, based on patient outcomes). Obviously the success of this approach will depend on the quality and quantity of information available on which to make decisions.

The sources of health information are discussed in the previous section.

There is now a much greater emphasis on information that could be available from general practice and may be consultation or locality based. The variety of practice information systems in use, however, has made this an extremely difficult exercise. As a result, a number of FHSAs have set up local information projects looking at developing the collection of high quality morbidity and risk factor data.

Other methods of collecting information about the health needs of the population included patient surveys. These look at patients' perceptions of health and local health services. Charity and voluntary agencies can also provide additional information about the services the public need most.

Assessing health needs must go hand in hand with an evaluation of the health benefits that services provide. Health gain is most likely to occur when the needs of patients, the demand for services and the supply of appropriate services all coincide.

Promoting health in primary care

Health promotion has recently become part of the common language of health professionals, but the concept of health promotion and its meaning to different groups has not been addressed. Everyone feels they should be doing it. Indeed successive government white papers insist it is part of the health professionals role. However, with no clear definition, no one is sure if what they are doing is appropriate or effective, and FHSAs have met problems over funding so-called 'health promotion' activities in primary care.

To GPs, health promotion may mean giving opportunistic advice to patients about adopting healthy behaviour aimed at avoiding ill health. To practice nurses, health promotion can mean, for example, explaining to diabetic patients how to look after their feet and eat the right diet. To the health visitor, it may mean exploring with a young mother how to budget for nutritious and affordable meals for the family or explaining why the children ought to be immunised. And, to the FHSA, health promotion may mean telling eight patients in a clinic to change their 'at risk' behaviour.

The first job for a facilitator may be to explore the concept of health promotion with the primary health care team in order to arrive at a workable definition understood by all, before health promotion in its widest context can be developed in primary care.

Although health promotion may include all of the things listed above it is not simply limited to providing medical services or knowledge to individuals about living healthy lifestyles. Health promotion aims to enable individuals to improve their health by controlling those factors which affect health. Factors that can influence health include not only individual lifestyles but the family, the community within which one lives and society, as a whole. Health, therefore, is not only affected by health care systems but by the government, social, environmental and economic policies as well as the culture in which we live, general education and the resources at the communities' disposal to express its needs and to develop healthy lifestyles.

Health promotion, therefore, is a general description for activities, which has the potential to promote health. It can include advertising, campaigning on health issues, legislation and social policy changes, control of environmental health hazards, health education, preventive health care and medical care. Health promotion undertaken by primary health care teams in Britain usually consists of health education and preventive medicine.

PREVENTION OF DISEASE AND HEALTH EDUCATION

In order to prevent disease, there is a need firstly to understand its natural history. In the presence of disease, an individual may progress from a 'healthy' state, through stages of asymptomatic disease and symptomatic disease for which the outcome may be recovery, short- or long-term disability or death. Intervention aimed at preventing disease will differ according to the natural history, and prevention can be applied at three levels.

Primary prevention

These activities are normally applied to prevent the onset of a disease or health problem. An example of primary prevention could be to prevent individuals taking up smoking, thereby preventing behaviour which could lead to ill health.

Secondary prevention

These activities are aimed at halting the progression of a disease once it has begun. It is based on early detection or early diagnosis, followed by prompt effective treatment. At this point the disease may even be asymptomatic. An example would be cervical screening where early changes in the cervix (precancerous) are detected and treated.

Tertiary prevention

These activities are concerned with the management of an established condition to prevent complications or further disability. An example would be the rehabilitation of a patient following myocardial infarction.

Primary health care is particularly suited to two types of preventive activity – screening and health education.

HEALTH EDUCATION

If health promotion is concerned with creating a social, political and economic environment conducive to healthy lifestyles, health education can be said to be concerned with raising individual awareness of the influences on health, and developing knowledge and skills to enable individuals to use the health care system appropriately. It includes developing understanding about the body and the effect of certain behaviours on health, how to prevent ill health and how to cope with health and disease. Health education programmes provide information, explore values and beliefs and develop skills to enable changes in health behaviour to take place. This is not about telling people they need to change to avoid ill health, it is about promoting individual self-esteem and self-empowerment so that they are able to make choices and take action for themselves.

SCREENING

Is concerned with the detection of disease in its very early stages so that early treatment can begin and thus a greater chance of cure. Screening, however, is not without its ethical dilemmas. Wilson *et al.* (1968) formulated a number of questions which should be considered prior to embarking on any screening programme:

- *Is the disease an important health problem?*
  Before embarking on an expensive screening programme some consideration should be given to the importance of a disease. This does not necessarily mean that the disease is widespread but it does imply that it may have serious consequences for a few individuals.

- *Is there a recognisable latent or early symptomatic stage?*
  Otherwise it would be impossible to detect before symptoms are obvious.

● *Are facilities for diagnosis and treatment available?*
It would be ethically wrong to detect pre-symptomatic disease
which has no chance of treatment whether due to the fact there
is no known cure or numbers are so large facilities are
inadequate to cope.

● *Has the cost of the programme been considered in the context of other
demands for resources?*
Services continue to compete for resources and screening
procedures are no exception.

● *Is there an agreed policy on whom to treat as patients?*
In other words the exact nature of the disease should be defined
before screening is carried out. There will always be 'borderline'
or 'less severe' cases. The decision about when to treat should
be considered before screening begins.

● *Does treatment confer benefit?*
Pre-symptomatic screening raises a number of issues. It is
fundamentally different from other contacts with the health care
systems which are normally initiated by the patient or client
who already suspects there may be a health problem. In
screening, the doctor or screener initiates the contact and by
offering screening *implies* benefit, that is, early diagnosis leads
to early and more effective treatment. If this is not the case, the
person may be worried by the diagnosis far earlier than if the
disease had been allowed to manifest itself clinically.

In addition to the above criteria, screening procedures should be
cost effective, carried out rapidly, and where possible by non-
medical staff. It should be acceptable to the patient, reliable and
valid, in other words sensitive and specific. Some of the most
successful screening programmes take place in early life, for
example, screening infants for structural or functional
abnormalities (such as congenital heart disease, spina bifida,
congenital dislocation of the hip, cerebral palsy, visual and hearing
defects) or metabolic defects (such as phenylketonuria).

The screening programmes that take place in later life, however,
are generally more controversial, for example screening for
hypertension, cervical cancer, breast cancer or raised serum
cholesterol. This is not to say these conditions are not important,
but it is argued that their detection could be left to case finding by
individual doctors.

3 The primary care facilitator

The development of the facilitator role

Pioneered by Elaine Fullard in 1982, there are now 305 (at Jan. 1994) primary care facilitators employed throughout Britain – 50 per cent by FHSAs; 14 per cent by DHAs; 26 per cent by joint funding arrangements.

The original 'nurse' facilitator role was established to help primary health care teams extend preventive medicine in general practice particularly in relation to CHD and stroke prevention. The majority now see their role as developing health promotion in primary care including providing advice to primary health care teams and FHSAs, training primary health care teams, particularly practice nurses and developing teamwork (National Facilitator Development Project, 1992).

HOW DID IT ALL START?

In 1981, Dr Arnold Elliot (a GP) was the first to use the 'facilitating' process to effect change in primary health care. By visiting his colleague practitioners, liaising with appropriate organisations and offering practical advice and support, Dr Elliot was able to assist practices improve their premises, achieving changes, where other methods had previously failed.

Similarly, Nancy Dennis in Tower Hamlets, London, improved liaison between the FPC, DHA and GPs and thus established channels of communication between the providers and the users. In 1985, Dr Michael Rope working in Kensington, Chelsea and Westminster FPC encouraged increases in 'group' practices (Allsop, 1990).

It was Elaine Fullard in 1982 who first used this method of working, to initiate changes in preventive health care in the primary care setting. The RCGP had published a series of reports on arterial disease which concluded that:

> 'About a half of all strokes and a quarter of deaths in men and women from coronary heart disease in people under 70 are probably preventable by the application of existing knowledge'. (Royal College of General Practitioners, 1981.)

They recommended that major risk factors for heart disease should be ascertained in patients under 65, and recognised the untapped potential of primary health care, which offers opportunities for anticipatory care as well as for management of presenting problems.

Thus, the Oxford Heart Attack and Stroke Prevention Project, was established with four specific objectives to:

- Test the feasibility of implementing the Colleges' recommendations.
- Examine the contribution a facilitator has in helping primary health care teams to extend preventive medicine in general practice.
- Produce a model which is widely acceptable.
- Extend collaboration between general practice, HAs and the FPC.

The results of the controlled trial demonstrated a significant increase in the recording of major risk factors for arterial disease in those practices that were helped by a facilitator (Fullard *et al.*, 1987).

The success of the model as a collaborative venture and its wide acceptability has been demonstrated many times now by the subsequent employment of facilitators in Britain funded jointly or solely by FHSAs, DHAs, RHAs or charitable organisations, and in other countries including the Netherlands, Australia, Canada and the USA (Cockburn *et al.*, 1991; Deitrich *et al.*, 1992). The numbers of facilitators in Britain have steadily increased over the last 10 years (Fig. 3.1).

WHAT IS THE PRESENT ROLE AND FUNCTION OF THE PRIMARY CARE FACILITATOR?

The majority of primary care facilitators are female with a nursing background and additional qualifications in, for example, health visiting, health education, teaching, a first or masters degree. There are also a number of GP facilitators and facilitators who have a background in social work, counselling, health promotion or practice management.

Although some facilitators have a specialist brief, for example, for HIV, diabetes or asthma, the majority describe their role as health promotion, training and teambuilding, with CHD prevention as a key responsibility. In a recent survey (NFDP, 1992) by the APCF and the NFDP, facilitators described their involvement in an average of 12 different areas of work. These included audit and development of policies and strategies for

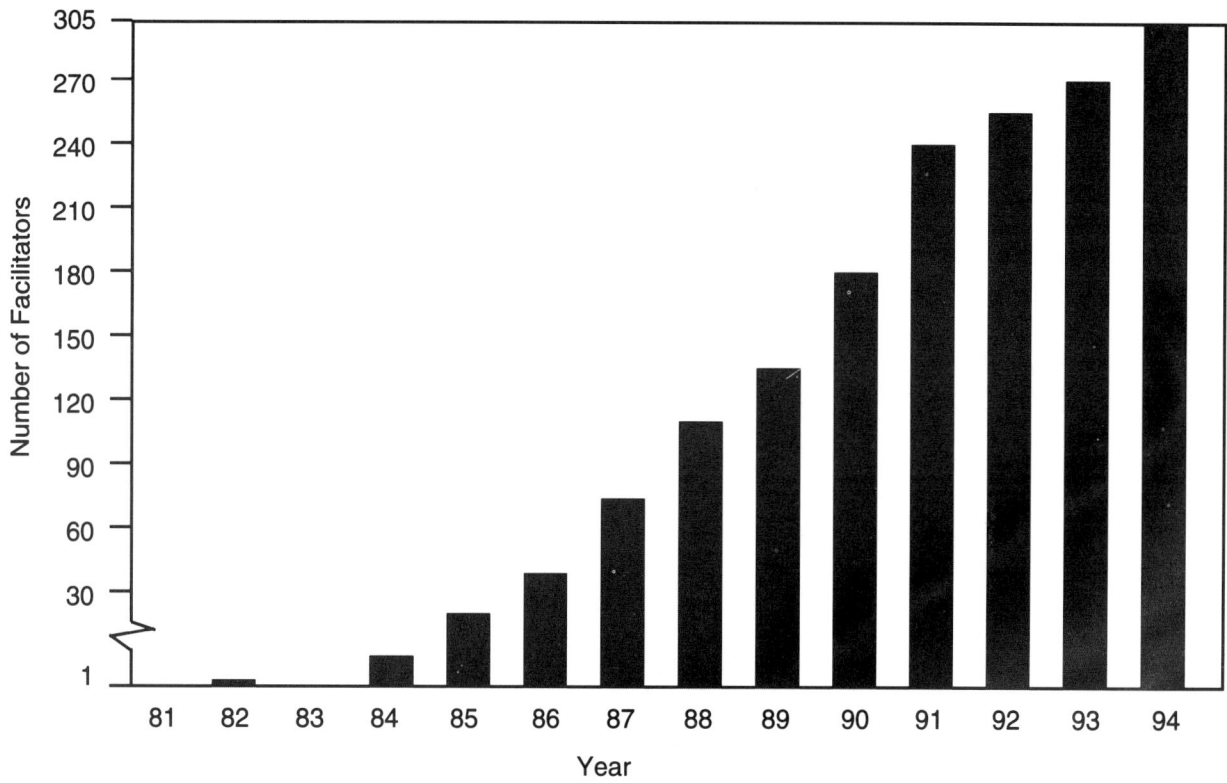

Figure 3.1. Appointments of facilitators

health promotion in primary care. The emphasis of the facilitators' work, however, is on the process by which changes and developments are made, rather than on specific topics or subject areas. The *process* of facilitation is to *empower* practices and individuals to develop quality health services in primary care. They do this by creating links between organisations and individuals and by providing practices with practical help and education to ensure changes take place quickly and painlessly. This may include providing examples of clinical and audit protocols and health promotion literature, organising training for practice teams or developing information systems within the practice. Developing practice nurse training and education and co-ordinating primary care team workshops has been a key responsibility for most facilitators. By acting as a 'cross pollinator' of good ideas between practices, the facilitator has become an invaluable resource to primary health care teams.

The facilitator role is still a developing one. A recent innovation has been the emergence of the audit facilitator in primary care.

Employed by FHSAs to work for MAAG, the audit facilitator uses skills similar to the generalist primary care or health promotion facilitator, and also focuses work around medical and/or clinical audit.

SUPPORT AND TRAINING OF PRIMARY CARE FACILITATORS

Support comes from a number of organisations. Resources are supplied by the HEA Primary Health Care Unit, the NFDP and facilitators' employers. Personal support generally comes from the employer and professional support from the APCF and NFDP.

THE NFDP

The Oxford Heart Attack and Stroke Prevention Project changed its title to NFDP in 1990 to reflect its national remit. The project aims are to enhance the provision of high quality care provided by primary health care teams by promoting the role of the facilitator and supporting all facilitators, regardless of their specific focus, in the development of that role.

The structure

The project is based in the HEA Primary Health Care Unit at the Churchill Hospital, Oxford.

The project supports three project officers:

- Project Director (Elaine Fullard).
- Project Officer (outposted in Division of General Practice, Leeds University).
- Project Development Officer.
- Researcher.

Posts are funded by the Stroke Association, DOH and HEA.

Functions of the project team

In order to promote and develop the facilitator role, project officers are involved in:

- Promoting facilitator appointments to FHSAs or DHAs who do not already employ facilitators. This includes:
  - discussing with managers the role and function of the facilitator;

  – providing guidelines for employment including job descriptions, salary scales and acting as external assessor at interviews;
  – speaking at conferences and seminars to describe and promote the facilitator role.
- Research and evaluation of:
  – the impact of facilitators work;
  – the support and training needs of facilitators.
- Professional development including:
  – developing links with professional organisations;
  – the promotion of training programmes.
- Training and support. The project provides:
  – induction training for newly appointed primary care and audit facilitators;
  – an ongoing training programme of skills training;
  – visitors' days (held in Oxford), for primary health care teams and facilitators;
  – attendance at regional facilitator support groups throughout the country;
  – a database of facilitator posts and facilitator activity;
  – resources including teaching aids and protocols;
  – bimonthly bulletin with information of courses and conferences of interest to facilitators.

THE ASSOCIATION OF PRIMARY CARE FACILITATORS

The Association was formed in October 1988 to promote the interests and views of facilitators working in primary care. Any facilitator who is employed in an NHS post with a district or regional brief to promote health in primary care is eligible for membership.

The structure

An executive committee is elected by the members to manage the affairs of the Association. The committee consists of seven elected officers, including the chairperson, vice chairperson, secretary, treasurer, members secretary and representatives.

Functions of the APCF

The objectives are to:

- Provide a support and communication network for its members.
- Give consideration to issues which affect members locally, regionally and nationally.

- Provide national representation of the Association to other public and professional bodies.
- Promote anticipatory care within the primary health care team and especially within general medical practice.
- Identify and meet the needs of members with regard to education and professional development including research.

In addition the Association produces a quarterly newsletter which is sent free to all its members. The Association is persuing negotiations with the Management, Science and Finance Union for future amalgamation.

THE HEA PRIMARY HEALTH CARE UNIT

This is a national unit funded by the HEA and is located in Oxford. The unit has strong links with the facilitator network both directly and via the NFDP. Its aim is to provide information, training, resources and support to primary care professionals in order to help them deliver high quality health promotion.

Primary health care team workshops

For some time now the Unit has supported and co-ordinated the primary care team workshop programme. These workshops, are intended to provide an opportunity for primary health care team members to develop their health promotion and disease prevention programmes.

   LOT, made up of FHSA and DHA representatives, GPs and facilitators, are supported by the Unit to organise the workshops locally and to ensure a supportive environment for primary health care teams making changes.

National database

The Primary Health Care Unit houses a national database on health promotion activities taking place in primary health care which is available to all primary health care professionals.

Helping people change – risk management training for primary health care professionals

In order to promote good health and to prevent ill health, primary health care professionals are expected to encourage their patients or clients to make lifestyle changes. However, within the constraints of a consultation lasting perhaps only a few minutes or at best 30 minutes during a health promotion clinic appointment, doctors and nurses have a difficult task to ensure their advice is focused and appropriate.

Professionals therefore need to be highly skilled in order to ensure they use the opportunity well and the outcome is positive.

In 1992 the HEA commissioned the development of a training course ('Helping People Change') for primary health care professionals in helping clients to change their health behaviour.

The training aims to develop the primary health care professionals understanding of:

- The concept of risk management in health promotion.
- The process of change and types of interventions that are effective at each stage.
- How to apply these principles to brief health promotion interventions about drinking, smoking, eating and physical activity.

The training uses the cascade model to ensure primary health care team members are equipped to deliver appropriate health advice. Facilitators, health promotion officers, community dieticians and others who are responsible for training are trained to run workshops for primary health care team members. The course covers the theory of risk management and behaviour change, session plans, visual aids plus handouts and other resource materials that will enable participants to run courses for primary health care workers.

Nutrition and diet

The Unit also provides resources, information and support to purchasers and providers of primary health care to ensure the development of high quality nutrition and dietary care.

Further information

For details about information, training and resources available from the Unit contact:

Tel: (0865) 226052/53 *for* National Facilitator Development Project
(0865) 226045/56 *for* 'Helping People Change' course
(0865) 226042/55 *for* nutrition and dietary advice and resources
(0865) 226054/95 *for* primary health care team workshop programme
(0865) 225587 *for* national database

Setting objectives and developing an action plan

One of the central concerns of the reformed health service is to ensure efficiency and effectiveness. This theme runs throughout all units and specialities, and all health service personnel are expected to evaluate their activities and describe what they have achieved.

This may take the form of an IPR. Many FHSAs and HAs use this system to appraise the performance of their staff and identify support and training needs. The process involves individual employees,

- defining priorities for the post and setting objectives within an agreed timescale;
- identifying the most rewarding and least rewarding aspects of the post;
- identifying areas of particular strength and stressful components of the post;
- identify under-used skills and those which need to be developed;
- considering how the employee could develop the post and what skills would be required for career advancement.

These issues are discussed with the manager and one other person of the employees choice, and action points are negotiated and agreed. Having completed the personal development plan a time is set for review. Each person keeps a copy of the plan and one may be sent to the personnel department. Some people have salary increases relating to achievement of their objectives. This is known as PRP.

Further information on IPR and PRP will be available from your personnel department. The following information, however, will help to clarify how to write objectives and develop an action plan for those who are not involved in IPR. It can also be used to supplement the formal review process and help you to evaluate your work more easily.

WHAT IS AN OBJECTIVE?

An objective describes what you hope or intend to achieve in the future and, in order to be measurable, should reflect *how* it will be achieved and *over what time period*.

WHY SHOULD WE SET OBJECTIVES?

Setting objectives are important for a number of reasons, including to provide:

- Direction – if you specify what you are trying to achieve, in terms of an end goal, or outcome, or objective, then the process of doing this helps to direct your activities towards the achievement of the desired result/objective.
- Benchmarks – it is only possible to evaluate performance if you have some standard or benchmark against which you can measure actual achievement. This means that you can use *objectives* to identify problem areas, and formulate solutions to actual or potential problems. Remember that a problem area exists when there is a 'gap' between the 'actual' state of affairs and the 'intended' state of affairs (or the way things 'ought' to be).
- Motivation – objectives can encourage people to contribute their best efforts to secure objectives they *understand, accept* and *internalise*.

It is possible to set objectives for an organisation, department, unit, or an individual.

HOW TO SET ABOUT WRITING OBJECTIVES

Objectives should relate to the overall aim or mission of your organisation, as well as your project or role. They will contribute to your strategy and action plans. The stages involved include:

- Defining your basic aim or mission. What is your job or project really trying to achieve? It may be helpful to look at your job description for the summary of your role. It may need to be expanded or clarified.
- Considering desired results or outcomes, and developing long- and short-term goals in the light of your aim.
- Developing methods that will help you to achieve your goals. Here, you should attempt to clarify the tactics you will use to carry out your work and formulate an action plan.
- Implementing your plans in order to achieve your objectives.
- Making modifications in your aims, and objectives, if necessary. Objectives can and will change over time.

WHAT CHARACTERISTICS SHOULD OBJECTIVES POSSESS?

- They should be related to areas of the job which are critical to the success of the organisation/unit/job holder. These 'key result' areas indicate priority, or the important result areas. Again, check your job description.
- Objectives should be measurable. Try to quantify them. If you state the objective as being 'to increase preventive programmes in the district' it is not specifying *by how many* and *within what timescale*.

Consider quantity, quality, time and cost.

- Objectives should be realistic and attainable, but contain challenging elements. You can also identify *targets* which exceed the objectives accepted as the relevant *standards* of performance. Targets are used in some organisations to motivate individuals to give their best.

TYPES OF OBJECTIVES

Routine objectives

These relate to those tasks which are an integral part of the job. They are always part of the required work activities. Use your job description for guidance here. An example is 'to meet with project team each week and report on activities to date'!

Problem solving objectives

These objectives are defined as those that are related to the actions which have to be taken to resolve the problems arising in the course of performing the job.

Innovating objectives

These relate to those activities which are designed to improve working methods or resources allocation and are consequently associated with improving some aspects of the job. Such changes can be long-term in their effects; they emphasise the need to find better ways to do things – constant *innovation*.

The list of objectives therefore should include some of each of the above – although hopefully not too many of problem solving objectives! Translated into action, these objectives will become your action plan:

- *Maintenance action plans*, to ensure that performance is maintained, and good standards are not allowed to slip.
- *Remedial action plans*, where performance needs to be improved.
- *Developmental action plans*, to develop aspects of your work not previously tackled.

DEVELOPING AN ACTION PLAN

Having decided what it is you want to achieve, you should consider developing a strategy or action plan. Your action plan is the method you intend to use to bridge the gap between what is happening now and what your goal is for the future. It has three phases.

Phase 1 (the investigation)

Begin by asking yourselves these questions:

- What has been achieved so far? What is the starting point?
- Is anyone else involved in doing similar work? You may need to liaise or collaborate with someone else within your organisation or from another agency.
- What are the barriers to achieving my objectives?
- What support or resources do I have to help me achieve my objectives? Do I need to ask for more?
- What methods can I employ to achieve my goal which are appropriate to this situation? Is there another easier, quicker, more cost effective way to do it?

Phase 2 (the decision)

- Having decided how to go about achieving your objectives, you will need to commit your ideas to paper. Some informal advice from a colleague may be helpful at this point.
- Establish the *sequence* of your activities. Where and by whom will activities be carried out?
- Prioritise your tasks, and make sure you allocate appropriate time to each task. The more important it is, the more time it should receive in comparison with *less* important tasks.
- Your action plan or strategy may need approval from your manager before you begin, especially if your plans are developmental. You should be prepared to give reasons to support your decisions.

Phase 3 (action)

All that remains is for you to put your plan into action, remember that you will need to remain flexible to cope with unforeseen events. This may mean some changes in your objectives and therefore changes in your action plan.

MONITORING YOUR OWN PERFORMANCE

Having set your objectives and begun to implement your action plan you will still need to monitor your activities at regular intervals to see if things are going to plan. You might find the following list of questions useful.

- Which parts of the job do you find most or least interesting?
- Which parts of the job cause you most problems or difficulty?
- How do you think you have performed over the last three, six and 12 months?
- Which things do you think you have accomplished particularly well in the last three, six or 12 months? Why?
- Which tasks could you have performed better? What do you think were the reasons?
- Is there any extra help or guidance which you feel you need to improve your performance in this job?
- Does your job description correctly reflect your major activities and responsibilities. If not, what changes are required to bring it in line?
- Do you still understand your main tasks and responsibilities, and how they relate to departmental objectives?
- Are any parts of your job unclear?
- How do you rate yourself in, for example:
  - problem solving;
  - communication;
  - technical knowledge.
- Have you identified a training need?
- Do you need to redefine your aims and objectives?

Evaluating your work

A FRAMEWORK FOR SELF-AUDIT

It is over 10 years since the original Oxford Heart Attack and Stroke Prevention Project began, when the impact of the facilitator was measured in relation to increased preventive activity in general practice. That evidence has led to the employment of over 300 facilitators around Britain and has initiated facilitator projects in Europe, the USA and Canada. Since then, the facilitator model has been adapted to other aspects of preventive medicine and there are now facilitators whose work focuses on general health promotion in primary care, some with specific briefs for HIV, mental health, cancer prevention or chronic disease management, for example diabetes and asthma. All appear to underpin their work with aspects of organisational development, particularly developing effective teamwork. Three further major studies in Britain have specifically looked at the role of the facilitator. The King's Fund study (Allsop, 1990) attempted to evaluate the effectiveness of the facilitator role and concluded that the most significant factor affecting the amount of change a facilitator could actually bring about was linked to aspects of power or access to higher management, whilst remaining independent. Studies by Fender (1991) and NFDP (1992) again examined the elements of the facilitator role and looked at what facilitators felt influenced their success, including the type of management which was most helpful and the content of training courses.

Perhaps as a result of the significant financial resources required to employ facilitators, their role is continually under scrutiny. In line with present development in health care, facilitators must be prepared to audit the quality and effectiveness of their work.

There is no reason why the audit cycle as described for medical audit, cannot be applied to facilitator activity (see Chapter 4). Bearing in mind that audit should be a simple process and should not, therefore, require the resources or skills that a research project demands. The first stage is to decide what aspects of the service a facilitator provides could be audited. Some of the questions you may like to ask are listed below.

Structure

How efficient and effective is the organisational structure in which you work? You may like to examine some of the following aspects:

- Time taken to reply to requests for information or advice.
- Dealing with telephone messages.
- Secretarial support.
- Your own time management.
- The accommodation, that is, is it adequate and in the right place?
- What channels of communication do you have with management?

Process

What particular activities do you perform?

- How do you decide?
- Are they appropriate. For example, which training courses do you offer?
- Do they meet the needs of the target group?
- What methods of working do you use. For example, meetings or consultation with primary health care teams.

Outcome

What changes have occurred as a result of your work?

- Changes in organisation with the practices, for example, development of protocols and procedures.
- Increases in preventive activity.
- Collaboration between different organisations.
- Changes in quality of health education advice given by nurses and doctors.
- Have you successfully empowered primary health care teams or are they more dependant on you? How do you assess this?
- What practical tools have you developed to help you and primary health care teams?

Having decided what criteria you wish to use to measure your work, you may have already begun to set standards about your level of achievement against these criteria. (Your objectives and job description will be helpful.)

The next stage is to gather the information. Do not be too ambitious. Begin with just one or two aspects of your work, for example, training courses *or* methods of working *or* office organisation. You may also like to do this with one of your peers, then compare performance.

Having identified problem areas, the next part of the audit cycle is about making changes. Although facilitators are skilled at helping others make changes, finding out what aspect of your work you need to change could easily be threatening for you too. The change may need approval from someone else, for example if it involves a change of office or change in focus of your work. However, with an audit to support your requests you may be more likely to achieve success! You should then set a date to re-audit, thus completing the cycle and remonitoring the effect of the changes.

4 Quality in health care

Quality in health care

The preoccupation with quality management developed from the commercial world – the USA and Japan led the way in the 1960s.

Although there has been concern for quality in health care since the inception of the NHS, the reorganisations of 1974 and 1983 more clearly defined the role of management in creating a better and more efficient service. The changes in the NHS have taken place as a result of the white papers which dominated the late 1980s and the early 1990s and driven by the government's desire to improve efficiency, economy and effectiveness. The concern for improved quality has not only gone hand in hand with ensuring value for money, but also with increasing accountability of health professionals, especially doctors.

WHAT IS QUALITY?

Quality has many facets and is not therefore easy to define. Definitions often rely on subjective views of what constitutes a quality service, and there has been a great deal of effort over the last few years, aimed at identifying the characteristics of 'quality' health care.

Consider the following definitions:

'Meeting the needs of the customer in a consistant and co-ordinated way' (Sage, 1991).

'Fully meeting the needs of those who need the service most, at the lowest cost to the organisation' (Øvretveit, 1992).

'The ability to achieve desirable objectives using legitimate means' (Donabedian, 1988).

'The balance of health benefits and harm' (Donabedian, 1980b).

Quality in health care then, is something to do with the organisation of care, the satisfaction of needs and achieving health benefits or improving the health status of the 'consumers' of health care.

Models of quality, provide a framework from which we can

begin to look more closely at the attributes which influence the quality of health care we provide.

Donabedian model

Avedis Donabedian (1980b) suggests a model for the measurement of quality which addresses three aspects of health care: the structure, process and outcome of care. These three components are nevertheless interrelated. Quality can be assessed, therefore, by examining:

- The attributes of the process of care itself (what is done to the patient and how it is done).
- The characteristics of the setting in which care is provided (including the location, equipment or treatments used, the knowledge and expertise of the provider of care).
- The outcomes of care, which reflect the impact of care on the health and welfare of individuals or population.

Quality is not about providing the cheapest possible care but neither does it mean that cost is not important. Quality is about providing the 'best value' for money, that is, the most cost effective and efficient care possible.

Maxwell's model

Maxwell (1984) suggested six dimensions of health care which independently have a bearing on the quality of care provided:

- Access to services.
- Relevance to need.
- Effectiveness.
- Equity (fairness).
- Social acceptability.
- Efficiency and economy.

Maxwell argues that the measurement of the quality of care must take each of these aspects of care into account.

Using both these models helps to provide a fuller picture of the concept of quality in health care.

WHERE DOES AUDIT FIT IN?

Audit was formally introduced to general practice in *Working for Patients* (Secretary of State for Health, 1989). It described audit as the means of 'critically analysing' the quality of medical care including 'the procedures used for diagnosis and treatment, the use of resources and the resulting outcome and quality of life for the patient'.

Since then, audit (and the audit cycle), has become a familiar and widely accepted tool for measuring performance in general practice.

The Donabedian and Maxwell models can be used to identify the attributes of care, which have a bearing on the resulting outcome. The audit cycle is the process by which these attributes can be measured. Implementing quality however also requires:

- Commitment to quality.
- Action, to translate good ideas for improvement into changed ways of working.
- The elimination of bad practice or barriers to good performance.
- Team work and recognition of the individual's responsibility to do the job well and to find ways to do it better.
- Continual measurement of progress and support for improvement.

Medical audit in general practice

Although medical audit has been a professional obligation, supported by Royal Colleges for the past two decades, it has recently become an increasingly important part of primary care. Medical audit is described by the Department of Health in *Working for Patients* (Secretary of State for Health, 1989b) as the 'systematic critical analysis of the quality of medical care, including the procedures used for diagnosis and treatment, the use of resources and the resulting outcome and quality of life for the patient.'

One of the central proposals of the Department was that all doctors should participate in regular systematic audit as a means of raising standards of care and to ensure professional accountability. Since April 1990 in primary care, each FHSA was to set up a MAAG to ensure that all GPs took part in medical audit by April 1992.

The DOH issued a circular, *Medical Audit in the Family Practitioners Services* (DOH, 1990) detailing the likely membership and responsibilities of the MAAGs. Funding for the MAAGs was made available to the FHSA from the RHAs. MAAG members were appointed by the FHSA after consultation with local medical committees and representatives of the RCGP. Although the MAAG is accountable to the FHSA for ensuring medical audit takes place in general practice, the health circular could be very broadly interpreted and a number of different models have been used to fulfil its objectives.

Audit is generally regarded as a professionally led, educational activity and the MAAG function is to 'facilitate' the setting up and development of practice audit activities. The circular also gives MAAGs the responsibility of ensuring that changes in professional practice occur when required and of directing, co-ordinating and monitoring audit activity. The DOH funded four pilot MAAG projects in early 1990 to explore alternative approaches to implementing medical audit. Liverpool MAAG successfully adopted a 'facilitation' model and since that time many MAAGs have similarly employed 'audit facilitators' to promote and support audit in their area. The facilitators may be part of a team of audit assistants, information and computer experts and administrators. The number of MAAG employees varies according to the size and composition of the area covered by the MAAG. Audit facilitators work in similar ways to primary care facilitators, but the main focus of their work is encouraging audit in general practice by practice teams. They can work individually in practices, or get involved in co-ordinating multi-practice audit and primary/secondary care interface audit work.

In addition to the MAAG budget allocated by the FHSA, audit facilitators have been successful in securing additional sums of money to support audit projects from the RHA. Regions have also made small sums of money available for nursing audit, which is on the increase in general practice.

As primary care facilitators help practice teams to evaluate critically the care provided to patients, particularly in the areas of health promotion and chronic disease management, there is an opportunity for both types of facilitator (primary care and audit) to work together. Particularly with helping and supporting practices in making changes. You may find it useful to contact the audit facilitator or MAAG chairperson, to see how you can work together.

WHAT IS AUDIT?

Audit is easy but has become enveloped in mystique. Generally accepted as a good thing, there has been a great deal of confusion and misunderstanding about what it entails. Certain key features characterise medical audit and are referred to as the audit cycle (Fig. 4.1).

All the steps in the cycle are of equal importance but some controversy exists about when standards should be set.

For the audit to be successfully completed the topic (identified problem) chosen should be (a) relevant to the practice, (b) an

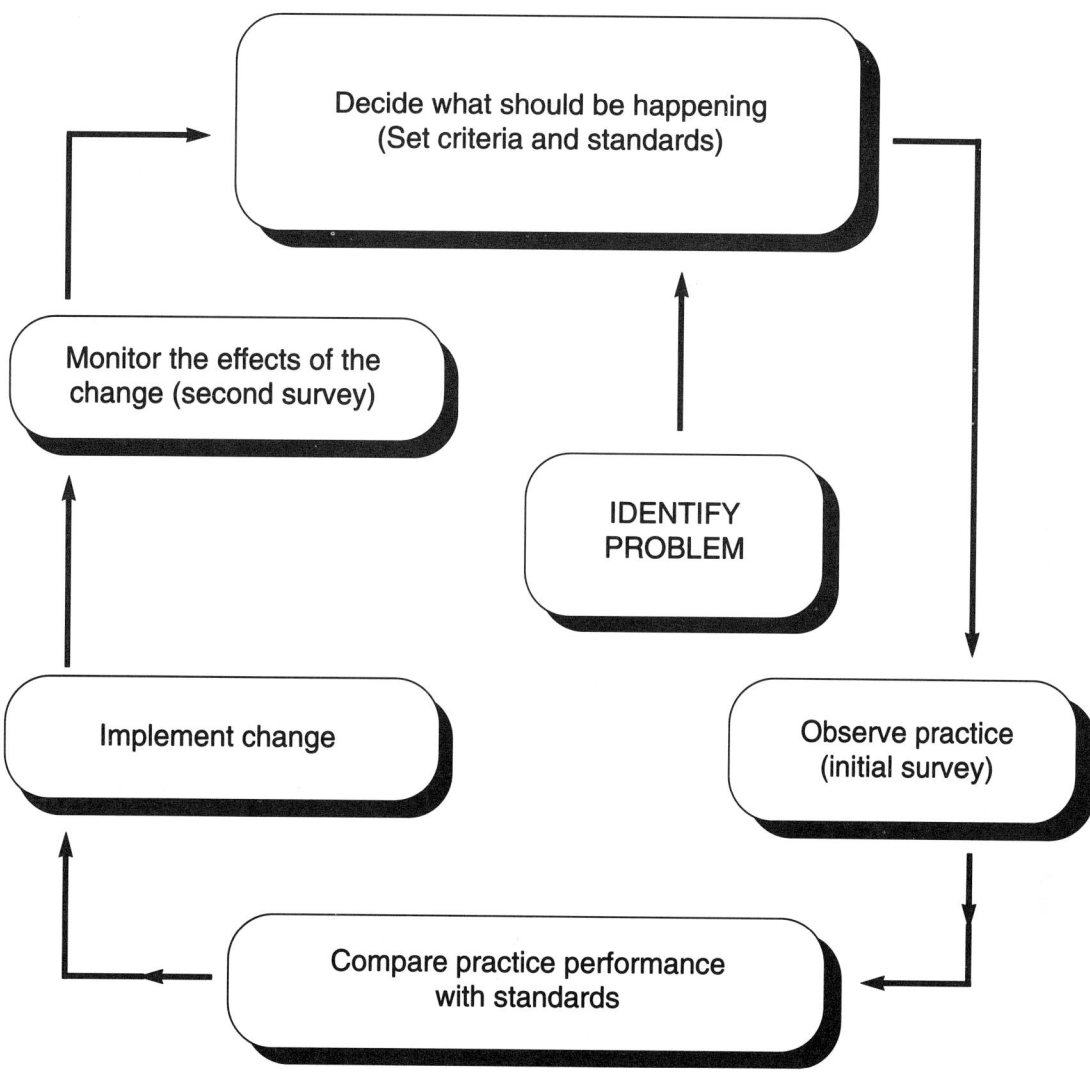

Figure 4.1. The audit cycle

important aspect of care or practice organisation and (c) amenable to change.

THE PURPOSE OF AUDIT

Audit may be used for a number of different things, for example, to:

● improve the quality of clinical care;

- identify and develop opportunities for medical education;
- enable resources to be used more effectively;
- help in the process of planning and development of services;
- 'monitor' and 'control' individual practices/practitioners.

MAAGs are promoting audit as an exercise in continuous quality improvement. This is much less threatening to GPs than using audit as a tool for monitoring and controlling practices even though managers may prefer to use audit to weed out 'bad apples'. They have been working hard to ensure audit remains an educational activity, ensuring audit information remains confidential and to providing practices with guidance and support in carrying out audit activity.

STARTING POINTS FOR AUDIT

Although some purists recommend that standard setting is the starting point for audit, gold standards are often hard to come by. It may be easier to get the practice to start by looking at what is happening rather than at what should be happening. Studies reviewing the current state of audit in general practice have found that:

- There is a fund of enthusiasm for audit (we should try to build on it).
- Much information is already collected but its use is poorly focused.
- Practices will find it difficult to perform quality audit without careful examination of constraints such as time, teamwork and difficulties with information gathering.

HOW TO DO AUDIT

Guiding principles of medical audit

- It should be educational and not punitive.
- It should be based within practices using practice teams (although the audit facilitator may be involved in co-ordinating district-wide audit and primary and secondary care collaborative audits).
- It should look at problems that are real to the practice.

Each practice (and facilitator) will need to consider a number of other issues

- Confidentiality – who gets to see and discuss the results of audit and how?

- The audit team – who is in it and why?
- Team decision making.
- Information – how good is the information system in the practice.
- Communication – both within the practice and the wider primary care team.
- Evaluation – how will the results be judged and by whom?
- Use of protocols – a number of 'off the shelf' protocols are available for use by the practices to guide them through each stage of the audit cycle. Before recommending these packages facilitators should consider how appropriate they are for use by each individual practice or how easily they can be modified. A check on the soundness of the content should be made. Not everything in print is of 'good quality'. (See also 'Protocol' p.62) The Eli Lilly National Audit Centre is involved in developing protocols of a very high standard that have been externally validated.
- Relationships between the FHSA and the MAAG – this is linked closely to the confidentiality issue. How will the practice gain confidence in audit without worrying unduly about the policing and monitoring potential?

Setting priorities

Practices should set their own audit priorities but may have difficulty in deciding what to audit. They can be offered choices which may be clinical or organisational. A starting point would be to look at national or local priorities for mortality or morbidity. Audits of smoking status, hypertension or cervical cytology are still very important. The audit facilitator should have a wealth of knowledge about which audits are suitable for 'first timers' and which have been useful or successful in other practices.

Information

Practices need to decide how:

- they will collect information for audit;
- it will be analysed;
- it will be presented.

Each of these three tasks is relatively straightforward but can be complicated by rushing in too quickly or by taking too much time to decide the best possible methods.

Standards and criteria

Trying to decide what should be happening (the first step in the audit cycle) may present practitioners with some difficulties. This is because:

● Traditionally standards have been set by 'experts', often from outside primary care. This can be very threatening for practitioners.
● Standards are concerned with looking at what health *outcome* is desirable and measuring outcomes is a new and difficult task for health care.
● There is some confusion about the definition of the terms 'criteria' and 'standards'.

A *criterion* of care is the ideal quality of care that is desired. Having defined the ideal quality of care, there are usually good reasons why that criterion may be very difficult to achieve. Therefore realistic standards that are achievable should be set. The *standard* then, is the proportion of events that fulfil the criteria. (See Table 4.1.)

Protocol

This is an agreed set of precise instructions (usually written down) that include the criteria and standards for managing clinical conditions or a feature of practice organisation. Audit protocols usually also provide some information on the background to the condition, precise information on how to gather data including data collection forms and summary sheets. They are becoming widely available but should be used with caution. Many have not been piloted or validated so may make the audit more complicated than it needs to be.

An audit protocol should:

● Clearly define the question the practice wants to answer. For example, an audit of diabetic care could include anything from how effective blood sugar is controlled to the patients' satisfaction with the organisation of the practice diabetic clinic.
● Not to be too ambitious but should attempt to set reasonable standards of care.
● Be agreed by everyone involved in the audit.
● Where possible be developed from existing clinic protocols or management plans within the practice.

Table 4.1 An example of the types of criteria and standards that can be set

All males aged between 35 and 64 should have their blood pressure measured at least once in five years.	90% This allows, for example, for changes in practice population and patients who refuse invites to attend.
All patients on anti-hypertensives to be seen annually.	90% Some patients will not keep appointments.
All patients attending health promotion clinic to receive *Better Health* leaflet.	90% Other leaflets or no leaflet at all may be more appropriate in some cases.
All identified smokers to be offered referral for one to one counselling or quit smoking group.	80% It is not always appropriate to advise someone to give up smoking. If a patient has particular health/social problems at that time, smoking may be 'helpful' behaviour. There needs to be some room for the health professional to make a judgement.

Outcomes

Although the overall objective of medical audit may be to improve patient care, actually measuring the improvement is difficult. It may be useful, therefore, to use either the Donabedian or Maxwell model to look at particular aspects of care. (See 'Quality in health care' p. 55)

Most general practice audits will look at the process of care because it is difficult to define the health outcome. For example, audit of a CHD prevention clinic:

- Preferred outcome measure
  - reduction in number of patients dying from heart disease.
- Actual measure
  - reductions in number of patients smoking (process);
  - reduction in number of patients attending clinics.

Choosing an audit team

As a facilitator you may be asked to offer some guidance as to who should be involved in the audit. This will largely be determined by the:

- topic of the audit;
- attitude of the practice to team activities;
- method of data collection.

All members of the primary health care team should be aware the audit is taking place, but key roles will vary depending on the above criteria.

For example, in an audit of diabetic care the team could consist of:

- The GP whose patients are involved.
- The practice nurse who runs the diabetic clinic.
- The diabetic specialist nurse or consultant specialist for the district (for information about the community or to identify the patients).
- Community nursing staff who care for diabetic patients in the home.
- The practice manager who may be audit co-ordinator or the main collector of audit data.
- Reception/administration staff who may be required to pull notes, provide computer information, etc.
- Chiropodist (if audit looks also at foot health).
- Audit facilitator/primary care facilitator, who may be involved in training staff, helping with data collection and presentation, and may need to co-ordinate and facilitate practice meetings and proposed changes within the practices.

Alternatively, an audit which involves a case analysis of one or two particular patients may, initially at least, only involve the GPs in a peer review situation. In other words, a team approach to audit may not be appropriate in all cases.

Hughes & Humphries (1990) describe in detail a number of possible audit approaches. The appropriate method to use will depend on the circumstances of each individual practice and scope of the audit. A checklist for planning audit activity is as follows (see also Fig. 4.2):

1. *Identify problem/decide topic*
   - What aspect of care is to be examined?

2. *Who should be involved?*
   - Arrange a meeting of the audit team and consider roles and responsibilities.

3. *Decide the criteria of care to be examined and decide what standards should be set*
   ● A review of the literature may be required.

4. *Identify the methodology to be used*
   ● Identify the target group.
   ● Decide the sample size.
   ● Design a data collection sheet (if appropriate).

5. *Carry out the audit*
   ● Collect and analyse the data.

6. *Presenting the results*
   ● Arrange a meeting between the audit team (and others), where the audit results can be discussed.

7. *Decide what changes if any need to be made*
   ● Consider priorities, be aware of time implications and possible barriers or resistance to change.

8. *Begin making the changes*

9. *Review the changes by reauditing (second survey)*
   ● Standards may need to change.

SUMMARY

An audit can appear complicated but in reality it is a series of common-sense steps (Fig 4.2). It is important that audit is 'owned' by individual health workers and primary care teams. As always, the facilitator's job will be best done when practices feel they have *done* an audit all on their own.

Remember the difficulties with audit, including:

● *Time.* Quality audit is time-consuming but worthwhile. Time can be 'created' by successful delegation and linking the audits to tasks that the practices were doing, or were keen to do anyway. Using a team approach with an appointed practice audit co-ordinator may be helpful.
● *Organisation.* Practices are easily put off audit. Someone in the team must take the lead on audit, otherwise practices are likely to feel overwhelmed. The audit method should be appropriate for the information systems in place within the practices.
● *Audit is stressful.* Not only is audit time consuming, the results of some audits may be perceived as threatening in the early stages to teams. Practices should be encouraged not to be too ambitious and to select a topic carefully.

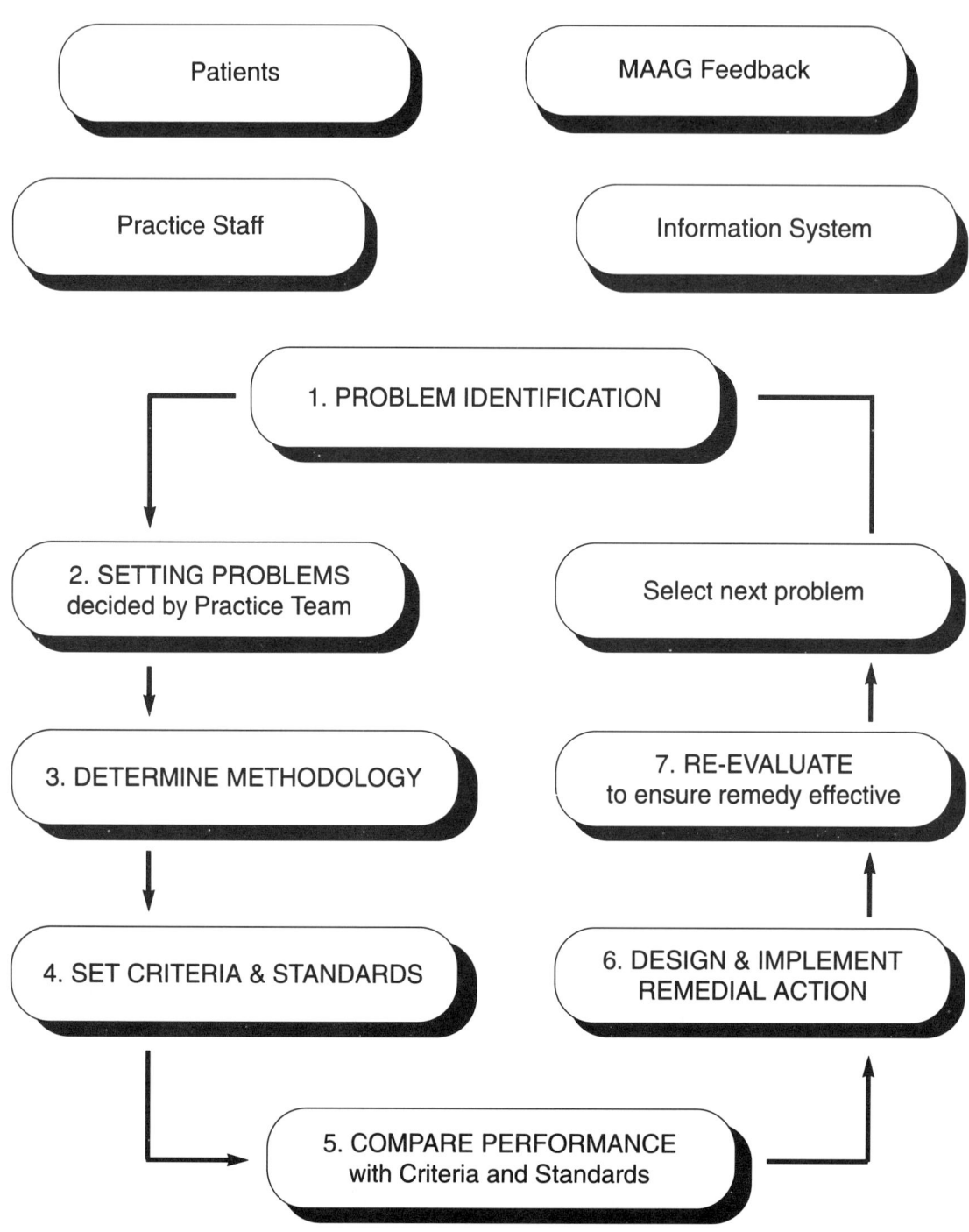

Figure 4.2. The common sense steps of a medical audit cycle

Some useful further reading is given under 'Audit' in the 'Resources and further reading' section, Chapter 7.

Auditing primary care health promotion activities

As a primary care facilitator one of your activities may be to help practices and the FHSA to evaluate health promotion in primary care. If evaluation has been 'built in' to the protocols used within general practice, collecting information about the type of activity that has been taking place may be fairly simple. In addition, some practices may have been systematically recording the short-term outcome of some of these activities. For example, the number of people who have given up smoking since attending a stop-smoking group or reductions in plasma cholesterol following dietary advice. The new health promotion banding arrangements specifically request some evaluation of the health promotion activities a practice offers.

There are several sources of information to help you with this work. Firstly *Better Living, Better Life* (Field & Henderson, 1993) offers an example of audit activities. The NFDP also provides a comprehensive guide (NFDP, 1992) to retrospective audit of patients' notes for risk factor recording. In addition, you or your FHSA will have a package intended for general practice to help them collect the appropriate information for each health promotion band. This was developed by the Department of Health in consultation with experts in the audit and health promotion field.

Do not forget that medical audit groups and audit facilitators may also be a help to you in this work. Many have published some limited protocols on auditing health promotion activities, which could be a good starting point for the practices.

You should remember though, auditing health promotion is not merely about collecting information about numbers of people attending clinics and risk factors identified. It may include:

- Levels of risk factor recording including, for example, numbers of 'at risk' individuals.
- Changes in demand for services,
  - as a result of identified health problems by the professional;
  - requests of clients/patients.
- Changes in services provided.
- Subjective health status of clients/patients and patient satisfaction.
- Changes in knowledge and attitudes of the target population.
- Changes in behaviour.

- Training and education of staff, for example,
  - courses attended;
  - needs expressed;
  - skills acquired.
- Organisational changes and planning services,
  - changing nature of services provided;
  - times activities held;
  - use of patient participation in planning services;
  - increase in co-operation and team work;
  - collaboration with other organisations, for example, local authorities.
- Types of resources developed within the practice/primary health care teams.
- Morbidity/mortality within the practice.

These are a mixture of structure, process and outcome audits and they can be applied to a range of health promoting activities including chronic disease management using the framework for audit discussed earlier. The important thing is to identify clearly the area you or the practice want to audit and to start small. One of the most important parts of the audit cycle is how the information from the audit is used to make changes. This is where the facilitators can help the practice to make the right changes and encourage practices to develop their work.

The Society of Health Education and Health Promotion Specialists has published a manual *Developing Quality in Health Education and Health Promotion* (Totten, 1992). It gives examples of possible outcomes for seven topics, including:

- Heart health.
- Substance use.
- Promotion of safety.
- Menopause.
- Sexual and reproductive health.
- Vaccinations and immunisations.
- Child safety.

In addition it proposes a framework for auditing health education/promotion services, which is useful.

Research

Can be defined as scientific inquiry or structured and systematic investigation designed to answer a question, throw light on a theory or solve a problem. Research questions are often described as theories or hypotheses and are expressed as sets of ideas or concepts, which are 'tested out' in the real world. All research must start with a question which most often arises out of normally observed events. Research projects aim to identify the factors giving rise to such observations and so provide explanations for what was observed through personal experience. Research can be either 'quantitative' or 'qualitative':

- Quantitative research is structured and deductive and looks for causes and connections using statistical techniques to assess the significance of evidence. A hypothesis or interpretation of what is expected is proposed, tests are carried out or data collected. These are then analysed to prove or disprove the hypothesis.

- Qualitative research is more unstructured and open to interpretation. It uses an 'inductive' approach, where descriptive data is collected and analysed. The researcher then offers an interpretation of the results.

Traditionally quantitative research has high status because qualitative research is more difficult to replicate. Qualitative research, however, may be used to identify particular themes or strands of enquiry in a given area, which are then subjected to a more quantitative approach. Important aspects of all research, however, include the sample used for the research, the validity and reliability of the data, and conclusions drawn.

MAKING SENSE OF RESEARCH

Every piece of research has weaknesses and strengths. In the course of your reading, you should be able to identify both. No piece of research would purport to be the final word on any subject, therefore you should not read it as if it was. Each piece of research starts from a different view point and so combining several research findings is the best way to inform your thinking about a subject or inform your practice.

Making sense of articles that present research data can be quite a task. It is expected that published research has undergone stringent examination to check the reliability of its conclusion, but this is not always the case. It is important, therefore, to ask a number of questions before reaching your own conclusions about the usefulness of the research. Some examples are set out below under 'Protocol for evaluating research methods'.

You can normally expect to find good quality, useful research material in the top journals, for example,

- *British Medical Journal* – not subject specific but normally clinical in nature.

- *The Lancet* – as above, also contains large international studies.
- *Journal of the Royal College of General Practitioners* – research relating to general practice.
- *Health Education Journal* – health education/promotion related research.
- *Journal of Advanced Nursing and Professional Nurse* – nursing research usually carried out in hospital setting.
- *Quality in Health Care* – all subjects with a 'quality' perspective.

Protocol for evaluating research methods

- *What is the research about?*
  - Is the focus or concern of the research clearly identified?
  - Are the theoretical assumptions implicit or explicit within the article?
- *Are there links with previous research?*
  - Has there been any other research into this topic?
  - At what point is it discussed?
  - Are the methodologies used in previous research discussed and evaluated?
- *Why was this method chosen?*
  - How does this method relate to the concern of the research?
  - Does it relate to methodologies used in earlier studies?
- *What are the aims of the research?*
  - Does the research aim to describe the context of the concern in more detail?
  - Is the aim to (i) test a theory? (deductive research); (ii) generate or formulate a theory? (inductive research).
  - Does the research (i) identify a range of significant variables about the research topic? (ii) identify relationships between variables? (correlation statistics); (iii) aim to identify a causal variable? (experimental research).
  - Does the research aim to solve a 'professional' problem?
- *How valid was the research?*
  - What features of validity were demonstrated in the research? (See 'Sampling' and 'Validity' below.)
  - Was validity explicitly discussed?
  - What criteria would you use to assess the validity of this piece of research?
- *In what way (if any) does the research inform practice?*
  - How far does the setting reflect your own professional environment?
  - How useful is it to you?

Sampling, validity and reliability

SAMPLING

Quantitative – statistical research

In quantitative research where the data collected will be subjected to statistical analysis, it is important that a *representative* sample is used. Statistical analysis in quantitative research assumes that the variables being tested are there by chance and not because of a bias in the sample. Therefore, an increased proportion of a given variable over that which might be expected will indicate that it is significant and therefore may be causal. The sample size will depend on the aims of the research and the methodology being used, but are best decided with the help of a statistician.

A number of sampling techniques for quantitative research have been devised. The most important of these are as follows.

- Random sampling – this assumes that the distribution of characteristics found in the total population will be exactly replicated in the sample population. The bigger the sample, the more likely this is to occur. This can be achieved simply by listing subjects and numbering them serially. Numbers within the appropriate range are then read from a table of random numbers until enough subjects are chosen. This can be done automatically by computer.
- Stratified sampling – this method can be used when the pertinent characteristics and distribution of those characteristics across the total population are known. The total population is divided into strata or subgroups and then a random sample is taken from each stratum. This is useful where, for example, age or sex differences might bias the result.

Qualitative – descriptive research

Other sampling techniques can be used for qualitative research. They should not, however, be used in conjunction with statistical analysis.

Analysis of qualitative data often describes findings by using percentages, ratios or proportions. It does not aim to test if a variable is more highly represented in the sample than one would expect. The criteria used to select a sample in this case may be convenience, opportunistic or incidental. Data are collected from a sample that is available to the researcher at that particular time. The sample is not claimed to be representative of the more general population.

Qualitative research often, however, combines the above method of sampling with what is called 'sequential sampling'. In this method, data are collected from subjects of a population until the researcher finds that they are receiving no new information and further sampling would not change the general direction of data already obtained.

VALIDITY

Refers to whether the theoretical interpretation of the data is real or correct.

In quantitative research, it refers to whether the research tools actually measure what they are supposed to measure, for example, is the Registrar General's classification of occupation an accurate measure of social class?

In qualitative research, it refers to the researcher's interpretation of the data, for example, are the conclusions drawn by the researcher a valid interpretation of the data collected?

RELIABILITY

There are two basic components to reliability:

- The *accuracy* of the instrument itself in producing consistent results.
- The consistency between different individuals taking the measurements or collecting the data.

A research 'tool' is reliable, therefore, if it is capable of gathering data from similar populations to get the same answers – i.e., that results will be 'consistent' if the study is replicated.

5 Communication and training

One to one communication

Much of your time as a facilitator will be taken up with meeting new people, explaining what you do, what you hope to achieve and challenging them to take on new roles and tasks. You should not underestimate the effect that your behaviour will have on the way others behave towards you and subsequently on the achievement of your goals. Your success may depend on how effectively you establish a rapport with the various people that you meet.

As your role is about 'helping' and 'supporting' individuals and practice teams, it is important to build trusting relationships that facilitate the sharing of information and enable you to offer more effective help. Helping relationships need to be based on:

- Genuineness – being open and honest.
- Acceptance – demonstrating an understanding of the knowledge values and beliefs of others.
- Empathy – having the ability to understand the way others feel whilst remaining objective.

Developing effective interpersonal skills includes giving attention to the way we speak, the content of what we say, how well we listen and how well we interpret verbal and non-verbal cues.

Although experience will have taught most of you how to communicate well, research demonstrates that making a conscious effort to improve your communication skills, will result in more successful and productive communication. Communication, is a *two way process* involving *sending* and *receiving* messages.

The words you use only form part of the communication process. The rate, tone, pitch and volume at which you speak all convey meaning. Likewise, *non-verbal* cues including nods, gestures, posture and appearance all convey important information which can influence the communication process. Effective communication, therefore, will depend on the speaker who must send the message clearly, the receiver who needs to interpret the message accurately and the environment in which the communication takes place.

THE SPEAKER

The following points will help you to communicate more effectively.

- Begin by finding out what the listener already knows – especially if you are giving information or advice.
- Say the important things first. People remember the first and last things they are told.
- Stress and repeat key points.
- Give specific information – vague general guidance is unhelpful. If you are unsure about something, say so and ask if you can come back with the information when you have found out.
- Sequence and structure key points logically.
- Choose language carefully and avoid jargon.
- Ensure communication is two way. Ask if the other person has understood and give them time to speak.
- Most people can only take in three or four points at one go – it will be helpful to provide a written summary or supporting material.
- Ensure advice is relevant and realistic.
- Try to establish a comfortable pace. The listener needs time to process what has been said. Try not to speak too quickly, however, speaking too slowly can be distracting to the listener and their attention may begin to drift.

In addition:

- Sit down (for anything more than the briefest conversation) preferably with chairs at the same height and positioned at right angles.
- Adopt a relaxed, 'open' posture (not crossed arms).
- Use gestures, such as nods, to convey agreement but avoid fidgeting.
- Speak clearly and evenly using pauses and changes in tone to emphasise points.
- Smile.
- Beware of too many 'ums', 'sort ofs', 'I mean to say' and 'you knows'.

THE LISTENER

As the listener you should be aware of both the factual content of the message and the way the message is conveyed. It is your job to listen attentively to what is said, to ensure your correct interpretation of the speaker's verbal and non-verbal communication.

Active listening includes assisting the speaker in putting across what they have to say. You can do this by:

- Responding with non-verbal cues, for example, nods and smiles and verbally by using short interjections like 'I see', 'Uh hum', 'right', 'really'.

- Paraphrasing what the speaker has said. This will ensure that the message has been fully understood.

- Summarising at end of conversation, for example, 'So you would like me to send you ...'; 'tell so and so about ...').

- Reflecting back feelings. The factual content of the message is only one dimension of a conversation and you may also need to pay attention to emotion contained within the message. You can do this by using statements such as, 'I sense that you feel very strongly about this area of your work'; 'I sense you are worried about the confidential aspect of ...'.

- Questioning may also encourage the speaker to put across the message in a way that you can understand and so will be encouraged to tell you more. Be careful, however, of the types of questions you use:

  − *Closed questions* allow only a limited range of answers, for example, 'yes', 'no', 'don't know'. They can be useful, however, to establish facts or to bring the speaker back to the point.

  − *Leading questions* put pressure on the other person to agree with the questioner, for example, 'You won't want to know about that will you?'

  − *Open questions*, however, put people at ease and show them you are interested in them, for example, 'How can I be of help to you?'; 'Tell me about it.'

Body language is also important and without saying anything the listener can convey to the speaker whether or not he or she is in agreement or is interested in what is being said. Egan (in Hayes, 1991) suggests the mnemonic **SOLER** as a method of remembering the importance of non-verbal behaviour.

S: Face the speaker SQUARELY.
O: Adopt an OPEN posture.
L: LEAN towards the listener to communicate interest and attention. Take care, however, not to invade someone's 'personal space'. In Britain people feel comfortable at a

distance of between 9 and 12 feet (3 and 4 m) if standing, perhaps a little closer if sitting for anything other than personal encounters.

E: Maintain good EYE contact, do not fidget, doodle, look out of the window or repeatedly look at your watch. These signals indicate boredom and indifference.

R: Try to remain RELAXED. If the listener is tense, the speaker will be too.

THE ENVIRONMENT

If you have an important message to get across you should, if possible, ensure that the environment is conducive to good communication. This means finding somewhere where there will be no interruptions – very often difficult in general practice. Ensure, as far as possible, that there is the minimum of noise competing for the listener's attention.

APPEARANCE

Finally, a word about appearance. Like it or not, appearance is an important part of non-verbal communication. A person's appearance can provide the observer with messages about personality, status and attitudes. You have the right to choose the way you dress and what messages you wish to convey. You may feel, however, that you wish to change your appearance according to the circumstances and what impression you wish to make. It is mentioned here only as a reminder that it does have a bearing on aspects of effective communication and can be changed if you wish.

Other aspects of communication including making a presentation and writing a report are discussed later in this chapter.

Organising a study day

Part of your work as a facilitator will include organising training events, seminars or conferences. This is likely to be the result of a need identified either by you or the likely participants, and may be to provide information, a format for discussion, teach new skills or simply to bring together fellow professionals to share information. The whole process will involve:

- Identifying and defining the need.
- Planning the content and method.
- Organising the event.
- Running the event.
- Evaluation and review.

IDENTIFYING THE NEED

Although you may have a 'hunch' that a particular study day/seminar is wanted, you will need to do some investigations to ensure your 'hunch' is right and the appropriate content and methods will be used.

Observation and interviews

Talk to a number of likely participants and find out exactly what they want. Talk to their managers, colleagues and your own manager, and test out your ideas.

Pre-course questionnaire

A useful way of collecting basic information is to send out a questionnaire. It is important, however, that it is simple to complete, the questions are worded well so that you get the information you require and set a deadline for its return.

Questionnaire design to assess training needs can be a very complicated exercise. If you want to perform a large scale study, it is worth getting further help and advice from other sources. Some useful texts are listed in the Bibliography.

Having a clear picture of what is required will allow you to define the need and to set aims and objectives.

AIMS AND OBJECTIVES

You will need to remember:

- Why you have decided to organise this event.
- What you want the participants to get out of it.
- What are the expressed needs of the participants.
- How you will know when the objectives have been met, that is, are they measurable and realistic?

PLANNING

During the planning stage there are a number of questions you will need to ask to ensure everything goes smoothly.

Participants

- Who do you want to attend?
- How will you advertise the event?
- What problems may be encountered by participants in attending?
- Is the date and time right, that is, does it clash with any other event organised for the same group? (Check the regional postgraduate centre.)
- Will they get released from work?
- Will you set any selection criteria?
- How many do you want? What mix of professionals?
- Is it appropriate to seek PGEA approval?

Co-trainers/speakers

- Will you involve others in planning, running or evaluating the event? If so they need to be involved now.
- How many speakers will be appropriate?
- Can they all make the date/time you have allocated?
- Will you be able to pay a fee? If so, how much?

Educational content and methods of delivery

- Are you clear about the content of the day?
- Have you made sure the speakers and trainers know what is expected of them?
- Have you discussed the methods to be used?
- Do you have a venue appropriate to the methods, for example, extra rooms for group sessions/workshops?
- Will you/the speakers prepare hand-outs to support the day?
- Have you decided how to evaluate the event?
- Have you arranged for postgraduate education accreditation?

Organisation, venue and equipment

- Have you found and booked an appropriate venue?
- Will it cater for the right number of participants?
- Is the equipment provided, for example, slide projector, overhead projector, flipcharts, video?
- Do you have a map to send to participants of how to get to the venue?
- What about parking?
- Have you booked refreshments and meals?
- Can special dietary requirements be catered for?
- Is the venue accessible to disabled participants?

Costs

- What is the cost?
- Will you need to make a charge?
- Do you intend only to cover cost or make a profit?
- Will you look for sponsorship, for example, from pharmaceutical companies, educational establishments?
- Who will underwrite the cost, for example, the FHSA, MAAG, HA?
- Decide to whom cheques should be made out – you may need to open a separate account.

Time

- Have you left enough time for planning and organisation before the event takes place?
- Have you done some advanced publicity so that people can set aside time in their diaries? If all details are sent out too early, participants won't reply or may forget about it, if sent out too late other commitments will have been made.
- What will be the closing date for applications?

RUNNING THE EVENT

You will be responsible for ensuring that the day goes smoothly. Begin by arriving early and checking the room is in order, for example, seating, lighting, heating, equipment. You may like to have a registration desk for names of participants and perhaps provide name badges and a course pack, including pens and paper.

Speakers should be met and introduced to the chairperson of the day, if there is one. They may also need help to set up equipment, organise workshop rooms, etc.

Make sure you have spares in case of disaster, for example, spare overhead projector light bulbs, flipchart paper, felt pens, blue tack for pinning up sheets of flip chart, and spare transparencies with pens. During the day you will need to be one step ahead of the game, for example, checking that coffee arrives on time, lunch is ready.

Ensure that everyone has an evaluation form and preferably completes it before they leave. If the course/session is PGEA approved, doctors will need to sign the PGEA register and will require their signed PGEA certificate. Speakers should be asked for the details of their expenses.

EVALUATING THE DAY

It is important to evaluate the event in order to:

● find out whether the day achieved its aim;
● improve the content and approach of future events;
● encourage participants to reflect on their own learning and what they have gained from the day;
● obtain feedback and improve your own organisational/training skills;
● provide managers with evidence of your activity and effectiveness.

You may like to design an evaluation form that participants can complete before the end of the course. It should include:

● A section on the participant's expressed needs and whether they have been met.
● The content, split into sections for the different topic areas, speakers and methods used.
● The general organisation including venue and food.
● An open section for further comments.

You may also ask participants for informal feedback about the event before they leave.

As well as aggregating the results of the evaluation questionnaire, you could use a number of other criteria to evaluate the event. These might include:

● The number of participants.
● The percentage from each profession attending.
● Speakers' views.
● Material produced with the workshops.
● Informal requests and comments from participants at the end of the event.

A checklist for organising a study day is given in Table 5.1 (p. 82).

Making a presentation

From time to time you will be called upon to make a presentation to managers, colleagues or your clients (e.g. GPs, nurses, practice managers). The presentation may offer an important opportunity to report on the success of your work or win support for ideas for future areas of development. Your performance can leave a lasting impression so it is worth doing well! Your presentation is likely to be useful and effective if you ensure that:

- The content is relevant to participants' needs and the information is demonstrated to be beneficial.
- It is clearly organised and presented.
- You give examples of real life situations.
- You use clear comprehensive language and avoid jargon, abbreviations and technical terms.
- You create some active communication with the audience, that is, stopping from time to time to take 'Any questions so far?''.
- You use good visual aids.
- You demonstrate enthusiasm about your subject.
- It does not go on too long.

PREPARING YOUR PRESENTATION MATERIAL

- Start by researching your audience, including if possible their status, background and experience. This will help you to pitch what you have to say at the right level and anticipate their areas of interest and possible questions you may be asked.
  Research has demonstrated that people's attention varies throughout a talk. It will be highest during the first 10 minutes and will drop dramatically to its lowest after 25 minutes. It rises a little after that and is high again for the last five minutes.
  If at all possible, therefore, your presentation should be kept short, 20 to 30 minutes maximum for an uninterrupted talk, and the most important parts should be made first and at the end.
- Begin by outlining what you are going to say, ensuring everyone present is clear about the objective of the presentation, and then at the end summarise what you have said!
- Present material in a logical order. Give each section a heading and subheadings; signal if you are changing direction, moving onto a different point or are about to make a number of points on the subject, for example, 'Now I am going to make three points, the first is ...'.
- If you want to demonstrate similarities and differences a table of comparisons on a slide or 'acetate', will be helpful.
- Do not include irrelevant material. It will confuse the audience and lose their attention.

Other practical points

- Notes should be used as a prompt. Do not be tempted to write down the whole lecture. It is better to write out headings on cards and use as a reference, thus ensuring that you follow the right sequence.
- If it is necessary for the audience to take notes, help by giving

Table 5.1 Checklist for organising a study day

Time	Activity	Action	Completed (✓)
12 weeks before	Find, visit and book venue elsewhere if not provided, e.g., Health Promotion Unit, FHSA, etc.		
	Book caterer or arrange with venue, including cost, times, and what will be provided.		
	Get/make map of venue.		
	Calculate costs and work out budget. Request sponsorship.		
	Arrange and book speakers Confirm content, venue, fee by letter.		
	Design programme and send to printers if necessary.		
	Send out advance publicity, e.g., flier, posters, advertise in newsletters.		
	Contact postgraduate dean and request PGEA approval.		
8 weeks before	Send invitations to attend with aims and objectives, programme and application form.		
	Arrange meeting with those involved in organisation or with training. Plan detailed content, decide responsibilities.		
4 weeks before	Send out confirmation letters and further details to successful applicants.		

Table 5.1 (*cont.*)

Time	Activity	Action	Completed (✓)
	Prepare handouts. Purchase files, paper, pens as necessary.		
	Hold second meeting with organiser/trainers to finalise details of content, evaluation form, etc.		
	Confirm with sponsor amount of sponsorship. Arrangements for display stands and numbers attending.		
1 week before	Check venue. Confirm arrangements for entering building, equipment, food and refreshments.		
	Make up packs (if used) and prepare participants list, name badges, etc., get 'spares' together (e.g. blu-tack, flipchart paper, pens).		
	Contact speakers by telephone. Check for last minute requests, travel arrangements, etc.		
	Check PGEA certificates and forms have arrived.		
On the day	Arrive at venue early. Check seating, other rooms and equipment. Label doors if necessary. Set up registration table.		
	Put up stand and displays if used. Meet and introduce sponsors, speakers and trainers.		
After the event	Send PGEA registration form and evaluations to postgraduate centre.		

(*Cont. p. 84*)

Table 5.1 (*cont.*)

Time	Activity	Action	Completed (✔)
	Arrange for meeting with trainers/organisers as a debriefing session to discuss evaluation and changes needed.		
	Write and thank speakers, helpers, sponsors for their contribution. Organise payment of fees and expenses to speakers, etc. Analyse evaluation forms and write an evaluation report. Arrange for payment of expenses incurred, e.g., venue, lunches, hire of equipment.		

them time and by ordering the talk logically. If you have a handout which covers all you have to say, let your audience know beforehand so that they need not be distracted by taking unnecessary notes.

● Make sure you can be heard and seen, if necessary stopping after a few minutes to check.
● If you are intending to persuade people of your view on something, ensure you present your views clearly, focusing on the strongest arguments. Anticipate and concede possible flaws in the argument and possible barriers to achieving your proposed goal. Provide, where possible, some practical evidence to help prove your point.

AUDIO-VISUAL AIDS

Audio-visual aids can be used to introduce variety, particularly if well presented. A few general points are worth noting.

● If your presentation is to be held in an unfamiliar venue, check in advance that any equipment you require will be supplied.
● Do not use any complicated audio-visual equipment without rehearsing! Arrive early enough to check, before you need it, how to work the equipment.

- If you are providing your own, make sure you remember things like spare bulbs for projectors, extension leads, adapter plugs, etc.
- If possible have a contingency plan in case machinery breaks down.
- Make sure the equipment you want to use is appropriate, for example, check the layout of the room and the number of participants. Although a variety of different aids make a presentation more interesting, too many can be very distracting.

FLIP CHARTS, WHITE BOARDS AND CHALK BOARDS

Flip charts, for example, are useful when collecting participants' ideas or when small groups have to report back. They can be used for emphasising or illustrating points. Flip charts have the advantage over chalk or white boards in that the sheets can be retained to be used or typed up later. You may also find it helpful to prepare some before hand if you want to illustrate a difficult point. Flipcharts come in a variety of sizes and are easily transportable.

Cautionary notes!

- Chalk boards - make sure you have sufficient chalk and a board duster. Do not wear black!
- White boards – always use the right pens, some felt pens will not wipe off.
- Flip charts – beware the falling sheets of paper! Ensure the paper pad is securely fastened to the top before you begin to write. Make sure all the legs are properly snapped into position. Do not try to write too much on a page.
- You may need to practice using these aids. It is a common mistake to write too small, put too much on a page or write in wavy lines.

OVERHEAD PROJECTORS

These are small, sometimes portable, machines that project an image onto a screen or wall. They are used with acetate foils which can be made in advance (to a very high professional standard) or written on by the presenter during the course of the presentation. They provide a strong focus for the attention of the audience. By using overlays of different colours, information can be presented very attractively and creatively. Their advantage over flip charts is that they are easily transportable in a file or folder and can be used time and time again.

Cautionary notes!

- Always carry a spare bulb, or know where you can get hold of one – they have a habit of blowing just as you are about to begin your talk.
- Do not prepare too many – it is very distracting to have acetate after acetate put up in rapid succession. Instead, have headings displayed and leave one acetate up while you talk 'around' the headings or the points you have made.
- Do not fill each acetate with too much information – your audience should be able to read it. Likewise, make sure the writing is large enough to be seen from the back. Unless you are in a very small room normal type size (i.e. 12 point) is usually too small, unless done in capitals.
- If your audience is going to take notes, make sure that by using a piece of paper, you only show the part you are presently discussing. If you reveal the whole acetate your audience will be madly copying your slide and not attending to what you are saying.
- Use the point of a pen or pencil to indicate things of interest on the acetate. If you use a finger and the acetate has been prepared with washable felt pen there is a danger you will smudge the writing!
- Once you have put the acetate on the projector, take your hand away! Any small movement you make tends to be accentuated by the projector and you will become aware of titters of delight from your audience as the slide begins strange gyrations across the screen.
- Make sure you position the acetate high enough on the projector. The bottom can easily be lost due to blurring or may not be seen at the back of the room.
- If you stop your talk to answer questions or dwell for a long time on one point, switch the machine off. The fan makes quite a noise and it will be a relief to everyone to have it stop for a minute or two.

AUDIO, VIDEOTAPES AND FILMS

These may be used to support a presentation but more often are used as an introduction or summary to a skills workshop session and can present information in a creative and exciting way.

SLIDE PROJECTOR

The slide projector is useful when giving a fairly formal presentation and can help to project a very professional image to your audience. A good slide will show a small amount of information and as with the overhead projector you should beware of showing too many.

Cautionary notes!

- Always arrive early to set up your slides before a session even if you have a carousal with your slides inside. You may find that the projector at the venue projects your slides upside down or that the projector is not a carousal feed. Either way you will have to sit and rearrange your slides before your talk.
- Find out if you have control over which slide comes next, or if you have a cue button for a projection technician to change the slide, likewise for the focusing.
- If you are presenting in a large lecture theatre you may also need to know where the 'lights down' button is – it does not look professional if you are knocking lights on and off all over the theatre!

Training techniques and skills for running study days

There are a number of techniques that can be used during a training session to stimulate interest, motivate individuals to participate and to make the learning process both fun and memorable.

Different situations, however, will demand different techniques, for example providing a straight lecture will be more appropriate at certain times than asking participants to become involved in group work activities. The methods used during a study day will depend on whether the aim is to develop the participants knowledge, skills or attitude. It may also depend on the participants preferred way of learning or the particular level at which it is aimed. The more complex the information or skill to be learned the greater the number of techniques that will be needed.

Research has shown that the attention span for most learners is around 20 minutes. This means that longer training sessions will have periods of higher and lower attention. Providing a variety of stimuli will help to extend the attention span. Some methods that can be used during a study day are presented here.

INTRODUCTION

The start of any study day or training course is very important. It sets the scene for the rest of the course by its tone and style. After the usual welcome, setting out the objectives of the course and eliciting participants' expectations will help to direct thinking around the topics to be covered and prepare the participants for the learning about to take place. Obviously, if there are a very large number of participants there will be less opportunity for feedback about expectations. This may also be an opportunity for you and the participants to get to know each other. This will be particularly important if you are going to ask participants to work together in groups.

You may like to use a game to make this session more fun. A number of examples can be found in Bond (1986), Collins (1983) and Danow & Bailey (1990). They are usually known as 'ice breakers'.

GROUND RULES

If you are training a fairly small group of people, it may be helpful to agree with participants certain ground rules (or courtesies) to be observed throughout the duration of the course. These can be written on flip chart paper and posted up on a wall for the duration of the course.

Some examples are:

- Only one person should speak at a time.
- Each contribution is valued.
- Participants have the right to pass or opt out of a situation to which they are particularly sensitive.
- Punctuality (both from trainer and participants).
- No smoking during sessions.
- Confidentiality – any disclosures of a sensitive or personal nature should not be discussed outside the group.

BRAINSTORMING

This technique is a quick and participative method of producing lots of ideas for use in later discussions. It can also be used when rounding up possible solutions to a problem.

You will need a flip chart, positioned where everyone can see it, and coloured pens. The facilitator invites the group to call out as many suggestions/answers as possible to the posed question. They should think fast and say any answer that comes to them, however outrageous. All suggestions are accepted without comment and written down. You can discuss the suggestions, group them into themes, priorities, etc., depending on the aim of the exercise. For example, 'Why do people smoke?' or 'What is the purpose of medical audit?'

LEADING A DISCUSSION

A discussion is useful for exchanging ideas and views and for swapping personal experiences. It encourages a two-way exchange between the trainer and the group members, and if carefully led allows *all* participants to contribute to the session. The technique often works best following some sort of trigger, for example, a video, role play or case presentation. Group members should preferably be seated in a circle on chairs of the same height. Although participants may have divergent views, care should be taken to ensure that no group member is alienated by the rest of the group. (See 'Ground rules' above.)

As the leader you should ensure that the discussion sticks to the point and consider beforehand how long you will allow it to continue.

At the end of the discussion, you should summarise contributions and draw out the main points or conclusions.

SMALL GROUP WORK

Small groups of about 3–5 people can undertake short structured activity, for example, an exercise, task, course study or focused discussion around a specific topic. This method can be used when a large group discussion would be difficult to control because of the large numbers of participants or when solutions to a number of problems or different solutions to one problem are required.

Usually, each group is given a specific task and one person is elected from the group to feed back the decisions or solutions to the larger group. Important points from the feedback are written on flip chart paper. Although the groups should be left to get on with the task, the facilitator should ensure everyone is clear about their instructions and answer any queries.

Participants should be told how much time they have to complete the task, and be reminded a few minutes before the end that they should be reaching conclusions. Normally 10–15 minutes is about right.

For this exercise to work well, it is important to allocate people to groups appropriately. For example, you may want a multi-disciplinary discussion or views from each discipline individually.

People who do not know each other should from time to time work with each other, so you may need to mix up the groups for different sessions. To get a completely random group together, ask participants to number off round the room according to the number of groups you need, for example, number 1–5 and repeat. Then all the ones go together, all the twos, and so on.

If the topic under discussion requires sharing of personal experience, for example, you may like to begin with people working in pairs first and then join up into larger groups after a few minutes.

ROLE PLAY

Role play is used to demonstrate real-life situations and increases understanding about feelings, attitudes and behaviour. It can also be used to practice inter-personal skills, especially responses to forthcoming difficult encounters, in a safe environment. Participants are presented with a situation which they explore by acting out the roles of the people involved.

People can be very wary and anxious about this technique and will need to feel confident and comfortable with the other course participants. It is not a test of their acting abilities or their competence in performing some aspect of their work.

Method

Volunteers are assigned parts in the role play. They may be given some information about the part they are to play or some indication of how they are to play it. You should stress, however, that role play depends on spontaneous reaction and there is no right or wrong way to play the role. It is meant simply to stimulate discussion. Those who are not given a part to play observe and give feedback to the players at the end. If the aim is to make people sensitive to feelings or difficulties which may be encountered in certain situations, participants should swap roles to experience different attitudes and behaviour.

Role play can be structured in various ways:

- Two or more people can play a scene to the rest of the participants and the 'audience' gives feedback when the role play is finished.
- Pairs, or threes, can work together simultaneously playing out the same scenes (this is often preferred by those who are nervous about performing to an audience).
- Groups can work separately with an audio or video recorder. The tapes can then be used for feedback.

After the role play, a discussion should take place around the main issues arising from the session. Participants can say how they felt, how they behaved and what they thought was happening. You will need to draw out the main issues for discussion and summarise what you think has been learnt from the experience.

Role play should not be used with participants who have not had the opportunity to get to know each other first, if there is not adequate time for discussion afterwards, or when some other more appropriate method could be used to demonstrate the points you want to make.

As the facilitator you will need to be supportive, be descriptive and not evaluative when giving feedback, and be willing to work with the group to solve problems.

GAMES AND QUESTIONNAIRES

These can be very powerful learning techniques. They are usually fun to do and helpful when concentration is waning. Questionnaires are used to focus attention on a new topic, make participants aware of gaps in their knowledge or show how much they have learnt, help them become aware of their values and beliefs and promote discussion. They need not be collected in as they are not meant as a 'test' and participants can work alone, in pairs or small groups to come up with their answers.

Answering questions around a specific case-study (often totally unreal, e.g., the desert survival game) is a powerful tool to practice negotiation skills, co-operation and collaboration.

There are also a number of board or card games that can do the same or can develop verbal and non-verbal communication skills. You will find a number of examples in Bond (1986), Collins (1983) and Danow & Bailey (1990).

A FINAL WORD OF ADVICE

Your local health education or health promotion department will have numerous resources to help and support you in your work as a trainer. If you are not confident to do it on your own, ask the training staff in the health education unit or your FHSA training officer to help, until you gain more experience.

Professional trainers are available and may be well worth the fee, to insure the training event meets its objectives. You may like to contact the HEA Primary Health Care Unit for more information about the 'Helping People Change' course. The course is intended to equip facilitators with the skills to teach practice nurses about helping clients to stop smoking, reduce alcohol intake, increase physical activity and make dietary changes.

Report writing

As facilitators, you will be called upon from time to time to write a report either on a specific event you attended, planned or organised, or as an evaluation or appraisal of the work you do. You may have to do six-monthly or annual reports and may also have a large final report to write at the end of your first term of funding, for example, after three years. In this case the report is likely to be substantial and may be used to support further funding of the post.

Although in the majority of cases a report is commissioned or requested, you may also be the initiator, if you choose to make a proposal about some aspect of the organisation or your own work.

Being asked to write a report, or even the thought of being asked to write one, fills most people with horror. This is probably because it is a form of communication not as commonly used as other skills such as writing letters, using the telephone, attending meetings and so on.

Not all reports are long, formal, complicated documents. With guidance and some practice you will soon feel confident in what you can produce. Hopefully the following information will be helpful.

A report is a written communication of information or advice, from a person who has collected and studied the facts to a person who has asked for the report, because it is needed for a specific purpose. Often the ultimate function of a report is to provide a basis for decision and action.

Although reports can be presented verbally or visually, this section is about WRITTEN reports.

TYPES OF REPORT

Written reports can be classified according to:
- Length (short/long).
- Tone (informal/semi-formal/formal).
- Subject matter (educational/financial/personnel etc).
- Timing (monthly/quarterly/annual).
- Importance (routine/special/urgent).
- Distribution (one to one/sectional/departmental/regional).

In all cases you should consider the RECIPIENT and should therefore include all he or she needs to know and nothing he or she does not need to know.

The information should be presented in a logical and classified order using clear, simple and succinct language.

PREPARATION

- Consider the purpose of the report.
  - Who is it for?
  - Why might he or she want it?
  - How might it be used?

- Draw up a timetable.
  - When is the submission date?
  - Do you need to speak to others?
  - If so, at what stage(s)?
  - What time is required to extract data/interview/observe, etc?
  - Set intermediate target dates for checking progress.

- Collect all the relevant material.
  - Notes, documents, visual aids, etc.

- Check the details.
  - Be ruthless and eliminate the unnecessary.
  - Add obvious omissions – it may be helpful to ask a colleague if they think you have forgotten anything.

PRESENTATION

Many organisations lay down standard procedures for the presentation of reports but there is no one *right way*. There are several *wrong ways* of organising and setting down information for others if *effective* communication is to take place.

The fundamental *structure* of a report consists of: an introduction, the main body of the report and a final section. Each part contains different elements of the report.

The introduction

This should define the scope and limitations of the report; refer to the person(s) who commissioned it; briefly describe the steps undertaken to obtain the information presented in the main body of the report; and include any relevant dates.

The body of the report

This should set out all the facts obtained during the investigation or period of work being evaluated; and present and analyse the material in such a way that the ensuing conclusions and recommendations are logical and warranted.

The final section

This should present briefly and clearly the conclusions reached and any recommendations, if necessary. It should also leave the reader with the final impression that you want to achieve.

Classification

The use of headings and subheadings will assist both the compiler of the report and the recipient. They will help you keep to the point and work in a logical way, and help the recipient to know where he or she is in the report and why.

There are several ways of using headings. Whichever type used, they should be logical and coherent whilst separating sections, they should enable easy transition from one point to another and they should aid cross-reference. Some organisations use a standard format.

The numbering system used can vary and, in fact, need not be used if the headings are clear. Generally, though, they are used to reflect the importance of headings and the material within them, for example:

I, II, III; A, B, C; 1, 2, 3; a, b, c; etc. OR 1, 1.1, 1.2; 2, 2.1, 2.2, 2.2.1, 2.2.2, 3, etc.

(the latter, decimal system aids quick verbal reference). You will need to decide which system you want to use and stick to it.

Whilst structure is important, the *language* and *style* in which the report is presented is even more important. It should be readily intelligible to all who are likely to read it and should not require great technical knowledge of the subject. Follow the 'ABC' rules of effective communication:

Accuracy – Check your facts!
Brevity – Be concise. Avoid ambiguity.
Clarity – Ensure clarity of expression through careful choice of words.

Memo/letter reports often adopt the 'first person' style, for example:

'As you requested I visited Practice X to discuss with the practice nurses the structure and content of the proposed diabetic clinic. During the meeting I obtained the following information ...'.

In contrast more formal reports (short and long) adopt the 'third person' style, for example:

'As requested by the Medical Adviser, a visit was made to practices in order to discuss with the practice nurses the structure and content of the proposed diabetic clinic. The following information was obtained from the discussion ...'.

This use of third person style frequently leads to awkward phrasing, stilted sentence construction and ambiguity. However, it is possible to be fluent, clear and concise – practice is all that is required, for example:

> 'I rang Mary several times last week' becomes 'Several telephone calls were made to Mary Green during the week ended ...'.

Sound grammar and punctuation skills are needed, too, if the document is to read as the writer intends, and is to achieve credibility with the recipient. Have a dictionary and thesaurus at hand to check the spelling or correct usage of a word. It will also help to avoid unnecessary repetition of a word or phrase, that tends to make the report dull or difficult to understand. Be critical of your own work. It may prove helpful to ask yourself these questions.

- Have I provided clear transitions from one topic/section to another?
- Are the paragraphs too long? Too short?
- Is the sentence structure of *every* sentence clear and grammatically correct?
- Is the choice of words effective? Have I used too many long words?
- Have I used unnecessary technical terms or jargon?
- Is the average sentence length reasonably short?
- Does the text read easily and smoothly?
- Are there any repeated words or ideas which are unnecessary?
- Has anything been left out?
- Have I failed to mention something early enough to ensure understanding?
- Have I checked the spelling of unusual words?

Text can be supported or replaced by visual aids but they must be purposeful.

- Is the table or graph really necessary?
- Is it linked to the text clearly?
- Is it labelled or identified precisely?
- Is it the most effective form of visual aid?
- Is its message clear?

Careful checking and editing is essential if the report is to be a worthwhile document and the initial timetable should allow for alterations and re-writing to take place.

Summary

To ensure successful report writing, *prepare* thoroughly and *present* carefully. Be prepared to do several drafts before you are finally satisfied with the result. *If possible*, get someone to give constructive criticism and, change anything that needs to be changed. *Finally* ensure the final production enhances your report. Have a look around at the reports you have received. You will see that by taking care to use good quality paper, and paying attention to colour and printing, you can enhance your report considerably with very little effort or cost. *Always remember*, that it is *your* report and, therefore, it is *your* reputation that is at stake.

LONG FORMAL REPORTS – ADDITIONAL ELEMENTS

The structure of such a report usually contains the following elements, but may need to be modified or adapted to meet the requirements of a particular organisation.

Preliminary pages

The generally accepted order is:

- *Title page* – this is the reader's first contact with the report so it is worthtaking trouble over its layout. It usually includes the title, author, date of completion and, sometimes, recipient's details.
- *Letter of authorisation and approval* – this is only included if requested.
- *Table of contents* – the contents page aids reference and selective reading; identifies the structure of the report, and includes page numbers. It is advisable to type this last!
- *List of tables and figures* – this list may be necessary if you are using a large number of tables and figures. It will help the reader to identify specific things of interest and it also aids the collation process.
- *Foreword/Preface* – this is generally used in large reports only and briefly explains why the report was written and why a particular format was chosen.
- *Acknowledgements* – it is customary to thank (by name) those who have helped in the investigation and compilation of the report.
- *Synopsis/Abstract/Summary* – this is a compressed summary of the purpose, conclusions and recommendations of the report. It is helpful to a busy reader and may sometimes be replaced by the 'Conclusions/Recommendations' sections, presented early in the document rather than in the final section.

Main report

The basic construction consists of:

- *Introduction* – should include terms of reference, and procedure.
- *Body* – should detail the findings and provide a discussion.
- *Final section* – should indicate your conclusions and may include recommendations.

Supplementary elements

- *References* – use of other people's work and/or ideas *must* be acknowledged in the text and then listed in the 'Reference' section. Any quotation *must* be placed within quotation marks (even a single word as it may express a major aspect of the originator's opinion). *Every* reference in the text and to illustrations should appear in the list of references.

  NB. It follows, therefore, that every item in the list of references must be referred to in the text or figure, and it is good practice for the text to make some mention of any reference quoted as a source of data. In addition, every figure must be referred to in the text in a meaningful way (i.e. not just 'See figure 2').

  There are a number of ways of presending references within text (Butcher, 1992), the one used in this handbook is called the author–date system. If a numbering system is to be used for references, the numbers should correspond directly to the order of mention within the text/figure. Whichever method is to be used consistency is important. In the references list it is important to include the *author*, the *title of the book or work*, the *date of publication* and the *publisher*, for example:

  Gowers, E. (1990). *Complete Plain Words.* London, Penguin.

  The use of footnotes does not preclude the need for a reference section.

- *Bibliography*. This is generally used when including other background reading around the report's subject area.

- *Appendices*. Appendices are useful when, for example, statistical data congest the main body of the report. The main text should clearly explain the part played by any material in the appendix. Make sure the numbers correspond.

- *Index*. This is only really necessary for very long, detailed, reports. Key topic areas should be listed alphabetically and provide easy reference for the reader.

6 Developing primary care

Managing change in primary care

Throughout the last five years, successive government documents including *Promoting Better Health* (Secretary of State for Social Services, 1987), *Working for Patients* (Secretary of State for Social Services, 1989b) and the 1990 GP contract, have sought to bring about changes in the organisation and structure of primary care.

The changes were intended to provide patients with better health care by offering a wider choice of services and by rewarding GPs for responding to their patients' needs and preferences. Many of the changes, however, have not been readily accepted by GPs who have, among other things, opposed the increasing emphasis placed on an economic approach to health care. They have argued that there is an inevitable conflict between financial choices and the doctor's role as advocate for his patient. Opposition to the changes were such that the 1990 contract was rejected by over 70 per cent of GPs in a postal ballot. It was nevertheless imposed by legislation.

Although primary health care teams are used to change, the recent pace of change has left some practices in need of help. As a facilitator and a catalyst for change you will have a unique opportunity to support primary care teams who are making changes, and to teach them the techniques to deal with change in the most effective and painless way. Successful change is complex and therefore planning for change is important. Planning for change involves being clear about what end result (outcome) is desired. Ideally, this may mean asking questions like, 'How does the practice envisage the way it will work and the services it will provide in the future?' Writing an overall aim like this is often referred to in management as the 'vision' or 'mission statement'. Most FHSAs will have a 'mission statement' which reads something like this,

> 'The FHSA will ensure that the people of Sunderside are provided with the highest quality family health care including general medical, dental and pharmaceutical services'.

There should be an agreed understanding among those who work in the organisation (or practice, in this case) about its purpose, its intentions and overall goals. This 'vision' and shared understanding of how this can be achieved are essential for change to happen successfully. Change takes place when there is dissatisfaction with the *status quo* and there is a shared 'vision' of the future.

The whole process of change is a cycle (Fig 6.1) and involves identifying the need to change, planning ways to make it happen, making the change and checking to see if the change has brought about the desired effect.

Managing change well, and sustaining the change once made is not always simple. It requires motivation and commitment from all involved and before this can happen there may need to be a great deal of negotiation and compromise.

AN 'ORGANIC' MODEL OF CHANGE

Tony Turrill (1986) describes change as an 'organic' process. The process begins with:

- Innovation – this may include new methods of delivery of quality care and innovative treatment used.

   Although there has been an assumption by some that before the recent 'imposed' changes, general practice remained static, this of course has not been the case. GPs have been developing a variety of high quality services for their patients including, for example, screening and health promotion activities. They have been attempting to be more flexible in their working pattern in order to meet the needs of their practice population and they have been carrying out audit of their work, so that they can improve where improvements are necessary.
- Ice breaking – an event (often external) 'unfreezes' the situation, for example, government directive to undertake new ways of working or internal practice problem.
- Leadership, vision and strategy – the combination of the above two points, stimulates leaders to come forward with proposals for change.
- Change vehicles/change drivers – once a realistic strategy is found and agreed, key individuals take on the role of pushing the change forward. New ways of working and activities begin to take place which shape the working patterns for the future.
- Refreezing – the different behaviours and methods of working are accepted and become the norm.

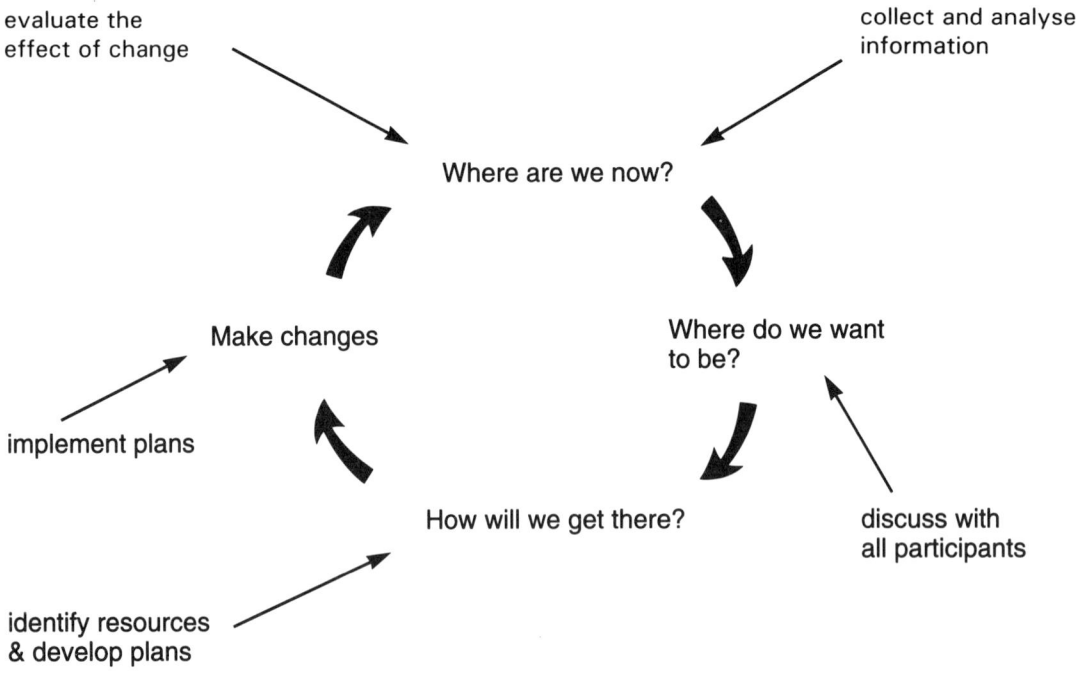

IDENTIFY NEED TO CHANGE

evaluate the
effect of change

collect and analyse
information

Where are we now?

Make changes

Where do we want
to be?

implement plans

How will we get there?

discuss with
all participants

identify resources
& develop plans

Figure 6.1. The change cycle

PLANNING OR PREPARING FOR CHANGE

Analysing the present situation

Before embarking on any change it is important to understand the present situation, that is, why do we need to change, what problems might we encounter along the way, who are the key people involved in the change, has the change been done before, and what can we learn from our past experiences? It is important to identify at an early stage all those who will be involved and to ensure that everyone understands the problem and the need for change. This will hopefully prevent resistance to change by individuals later on.

Individuals react to change in different ways and therefore may behave in different ways. Six possible roles have been identified:

- Generating ideas for change.
- Selling ideas for change.
- Sustaining change.

These roles are essentially positive and embody a personal commitment to change.

- Consuming change.

- Obstructing change.
- Ignoring change.

These three are essentially negative and infer no ownership of the proposed change. Consuming the change means that the person accepts it and supports it in a passive way but relies on others to be the prime mover. Obstructing the change is when someone overtly *or* covertly puts barriers in the way to prevent change occurring. Ignoring the change means that change is seen as peripheral to the persons' own activities and is too distant for their concern.

A successful team will predominantly include members who are skilled to assume the first three roles, although at times they too may be passive consumers of change. It is those who continually adopt the last three roles that are likely to obstruct the changes.

One's attitude to change may depend on past experience and may also be influenced by present motives and priorities. Perceptions of how the change will affect, for example, the individual's status and reputation, self image, finance, other commitments or work load all influence how individuals react to change.

Other possible barriers within a practice may include one or more of the following:

- The structure of the practice, for example, premises, practice area, size.
- Personnel, for example, number, skills.
- Lack of or perceived lack of time.
- Finance.
- Expectations – individual and those of the practice team, or external expectations, for example, the patients, the FHSA, government.
- Whether the change is imposed or has been identified as a result of an internal problem.

Research in management has demonstrated that successful change will only happen if there is sufficient 'slack' to cope with the change. This implies that resources must be free to enable the change to take place. Making changes, therefore, may also involve creating the 'slack', that is, using more money, finding extra staff.

One way of looking at possible barriers, and enablers of, change is by using a 'force field analysis'. It can be used by individuals, that is, as a facilitator trying to see why changes are not taking place or are making very slow progress, or by groups planning for change.

The technique requires a description of the situation as it is now and a vision of the future. Then a list is drawn up of the forces driving the change and a list of the barriers or restraining forces opposing it. These may include forces concerned with personal, interpersonal, intergroup, managerial, organisational, technological and environmental factors. The restraining and driving forces are listed down each side of the paper. A line down the centre represents the *status quo*. The strength of each force should be represented by an arrow which can be drawn with various degrees of thickness. An example is given in Fig. 6.2.

The aim is then to work on lessening the restraining forces. Putting extra pressure on the driving forces may only generate new opposing ones.

This model can give an insight into whether the practice is ready for change and what actions you or the practice may need to take to prepare it for change, for example, find extra resources (staff, finance, space, etc.), who or what will support the change and who or what will hinder the success of the change. Facilitating change in general practice should involve helping to minimise restraining forces to change as well as encouraging changes to take place.

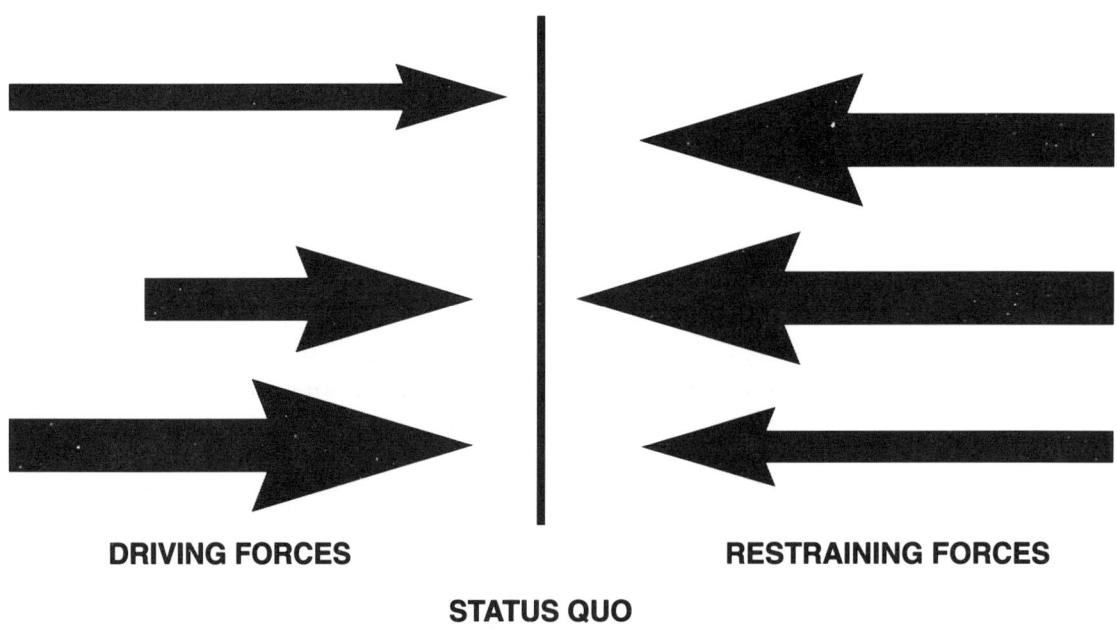

DRIVING FORCES   **RESTRAINING FORCES**

STATUS QUO

Figure 6.2. Force field analysis

Successful changes depend on clarity of purpose, a widely shared vision of the future, a set of agreed beliefs, values and principles which govern the way people operate. Negotiation with all the 'stakeholders' (all those who are affected by the change) will ensure ownership of the change and is more likely to result in success.

IMPLEMENTING THE CHANGE

Defining and agreeing goals

Sharing a vision for the future also means defining and coming to agreement about the objectives that will help to achieve the change. Reaching a consensus may require some compromise, before everyone begins to work together. The ease with which this is achieved also depends on how decisions are normally reached within the practice. (See 'Making decisions', p. 112.)

Working towards a 'consensus' decision will give individuals the opportunity to voice their opinions and concerns and prevent blocks and disruptions later on. If the change solves a problem for everyone then consensus will be reached more easily.

Aims and objectives should always be written down so that achievements can be assessed later on.

Developing a strategy

All possible methods of achieving the change should be explored. This may involve some research into the particular focus of change. For example, computerising the practice will involve negotiating with a number of suppliers, discussing the range and suitability of different software programmes and exploring such things as cost and training. Starting a stop-smoking group may involve examining the literature to discover the best methods, finding out what can be supplied from the local health education unit, finding out what format patients would like and checking about funding from the FHSA. Armed with all the relevant information, and having presented and discussed the possible choices, the practice can then set about agreeing tasks and responsibilities.

Most changes are best tackled as a team activity. This way, the workload and responsibility is shared, each member feels valued for his or her contribution and has a keen interest in seeing that the change works. Each person's particular skills can be used appropriately and selecting a co-ordinator or 'transition leader' may be helpful in ensuring things go to plan and the timetable is adhered to. Realistic timescales should be set and as far as possible adhered to, although there may be factors outside the control of the practice which can either speed up or slow down progress.

How do we know when we have arrived?

It is important in the planning stages to ensure that criteria for success are defined. Ultimately, they will lead to achievement of the overall aim or outcome but there may be a variety of steps along the way or peripheral criteria which are equally important. Each should have a clear timescale.

As change is often a complex process and one change often leads to another, it can be difficult to say with certainty that one change has begun and another ended. Defining a specific time period will be helpful so that progress can be measured up to that point. To ensure that changes are sustained it may be necessary to change or develop practice policies and guidelines. These will ensure that the change is not forgotten and staff members are clear about the new methods of working. This is the period when 'refreezing' occurs, the change is allowed to settle in and the new ways of working become the norm.

Every change should include a full evaluation or review. It should look back at the change and the process of change and ask a number of questions.

- Aims
  - Have we achieved what we wanted? If not, why not? Should our aims have been different?

- Methods
  - Was the method we used appropriate, the best use of time, money, people?

- Cost/benefit
  - Has the change been successful and beneficial?
  - Is the result better than if we hadn't made the change?

- Other effects
  - Has there been any 'spin offs' like other beneficial effects? For example, has it improved teamwork, communication within the practice, staff morale?
  - Who in the end were the 'winners' and who the 'losers'?
  - What lessons have we learnt?

Finally, any achievement, however small, requires acknowledgement and praise. We are often so busy moving onto the next project that hard work goes unrecognised and taken for granted. Celebrating success will build team cohesiveness, reassert the teams ability to succeed and motivate the team for future development. As a facilitator, if you have done your job well, the team will feel better able to cope with change more effectively. You must recognise when to let go. Your fulfilment should come from witnessing the developments you have successfully facilitated, even though you may not be given full recognition for the part you have played.

Teams and teambuilding

As a primary care facilitator, you are likely to come into contact with a number of different teams. For some of these teams, you will function as a team member, for example, a team of primary care facilitators, a health promotion team, a medical/nursing team or an FHSA management team. You are also likely to have a specific remit to develop the primary health care team and other teams with which you work, to enhance their team effectiveness. It is important, therefore, in order to work most effectively with teams and to function well as a team member, that you have an understanding of the process of team working.

WHAT IS A TEAM?

Some definitions:

> 'A team is a collection of individuals who have an explicit reason for working together, and are in need of each others' abilities and skills'. (NHS Training Authority.)
> 'Teams are groups of people who co-operate to carry out a joint task'. (Argyle, 1973.)
> '... a team is a group of people who make different contributions towards the achievement of a common goal'. (Pritchard, 1981.)

Teams that work well display a number of important characteristics (Gilmore *et al.*, 1974):

- A common purpose – accepted and understood by all team members.
- A clear understanding by each team member of their roles, function and responsibility.
- A shared knowledge and respect of other members' roles, function, skills and responsibility.
- Pooling of knowledge, skills and resources and shared responsibility for the outcome.
- Capable of working as an autonomous group of people.

There is, however, no one team structure or process which is perfect for every situation. A team will develop over time, providing the above issues are observed and team members communicate regularly and in a meaningful way. Research has demonstrated that effective teamwork can increase productivity, improve the quality of the end result, be cost-effective in time and resources and can enhance working relationships.

It requires motivation from all team members to be flexible and co-operative and to communicate well, and time and effort needs to be put into careful planning of team activities.

TEAM MEMBERSHIP AND TEAM ROLES

Deciding the purpose of a team and establishing team objectives will help to clarify the membership of the team.

By establishing the exact skills and expertise needed to accomplish the team task, it should be possible to identify which roles are required. Although each member is likely to have a professional (expert) role within a team, roles may change according to the team task and one person may assume a number of roles throughout the life of the group. Research has demonstrated that there are two types of function group members perform in order that the group functions well. These have been described as 'task' and 'maintenance' functions. They are both contrasting and complementary.

Individuals involved in the 'task' functions, assume responsibility for getting the 'task done'. Individuals who play a 'maintenance' function, are concerned with the group process and essentially maintain the right atmosphere or environment within the group, in order to allow the objectives of the group to be met. Without the 'maintenance' function, the groups' ability to work as a co-operative unit would not be achieved. Individuals may adopt either of these functions at any particular time.

Adair (1986) also argues that group members have an 'individual' need for personal fulfilment. It is this need which motivates members to join the group and contribute to the joint task. A group can be thought of as an 'embryonic' team. Thus a team is a more highly developed effective group.

Studies of the way individuals work in groups have demonstrated a number of key elements to these functions.

TASK FUNCTIONS

Initiator

The person who starts things off or puts new impetus into the group when a new way of working seems necessary. For example,

'We'll begin by ...', 'Maybe what we should do now is ...', 'There is a new way of looking at this ...'.

Clarifier

This is the person who teases the precise meaning out of general statements, makes connections between individual contributions.

Information giving

The person who provides additional new information. This may, for example, be technical or relate to the understanding of the nature of a task.

Questioning

This person may challenge assumptions the group is making. For example, 'Is this the only option open?', 'How do you think this will affect ...?'.

Summarising

This person pulls various contributions together in a conclusive manner. It can allow the group to reflect on its progress and sets a baseline for the next phase of work.

MAINTENANCE FUNCTIONS

Supporter

This can be done verbally, by acknowledging and including a person or their contribution. For example, 'Yes, I think that's a really good point', or non-verbally (by head nodding, eye contact or smiling).

Light relief

When the tension is high, humour gives people the chance to laugh and let off steam. It should not be used in a destructive way.

Sharing experiences

Sharing personal experiences about the issues being discussed encourages the group to relate at a deeper level. It creates an atmosphere of 'realness' in the situation.

Process observers

This means taking a step back from what is happening on the surface and examining how people relate to one another and why they behave in that way. For example, 'I notice that there are some who haven't as yet had the chance to speak', 'I wonder if we need to look at why we're going round in circles'.

Other studies have revealed that a mix of several roles which demonstrate clearly distinguishable characteristics can be found in effective teams.

TEAM ROLE CLASSIFICATION (Belbin, 1981)

- Chairperson – resides over the team and co-ordinates its efforts. Need not be brilliant or creative. It is more important that they should be disciplined, focused and balanced, a good listener and talker, effective at working through others.
- Shaper – highly strung, outgoing and dominant, this person is the task leader, demonstrating a drive and passion for completing the task. May become irritable and impatient, but provides a spur to action.
- Plant – may be introverted, but is intellectually dominant. The ideas person, capable of divergent and imaginative thinking but may be careless about details or finishing.
- Evaluator – intelligent but in an analytical rather than creative way. They are able to analyse ideas accurately and assess their feasibility in relation to a host of factors and variables. May be aloof from the team, more at home with data than people.
- Investigator – extrovert, sociable and relaxed. Brings new contracts, ideas and developments to the group, acts as the liaison officer or diplomat for the group, making useful contacts with the outside world. Needs the group to pick up contributions.
- Worker – practical organiser, turning team decisions into action in the form of manageable tasks. Methodical, trustworthy and efficient. Does not lead but excels in administration.
- Team worker – holds the team together by supporting others, listening, encouraging and harmonising. Likeable and popular, often remains unnoticed when present, but missed when absent.
- Finisher – without this person, the team might never meet its deadlines. Checks details and urges others on, trying to overcome snags that arise. An important role but because it involves an element of pressure and chasing up, it is not always popular.

Too many of one role type will 'unbalance' a team and too few of one type will result in uncompleted tasks. In a small team therefore, one member may need to adopt more than one role. In real life of course, it is not always possible to pick the team members according to their skills or particular strengths. An understanding of the roles team members play, however, will help you to assess the team, diagnose possible problems and develop the strengths of team members, to improve team performance. It is helpful for team members to reflect on the role they play and be aware of the contribution other team members provide.

There are a number of other factors which influence how the team works together, some of which are unconscious and irrational, for example, number of people in the team, whether they were previously known to one another, whether they are part of the team through their own choice or if they have been forced into it, leadership style, the comfort or lack of comfort of the environment, individual hidden agendas or how the group is made up in relation to gender, age and amount of experience.

These factors will affect the group's pattern of development – a process sometimes described as group life. Researchers who have observed the way groups work have described the process by using 'models'. No one model provides a 'right' explanation but they can be useful in helping us understand the complex interactions between group members. One such model is Tuckman's model of group life (Argyle, 1973).

TUCKMAN'S MODEL OF GROUP LIFE

The group is described as progressing through four stages either sequentially or moving back and forth from one stage to another (Argyle, 1973).

- Forming – testing out what behaviours are acceptable and what the norms of the group will be. How supportive, critical, serious or humorous will the group be. Very little open exchange of views take place at this stage.
- Storming – atmosphere of conflict, rebellion with leader, polarisation of opinion, resistance to control. Sense of task being impossible. The task, however, is at this stage beginning to be taken seriously and individuals are working out the personal implications.
- Norming – at this stage group cohesion develops and norms for the group emerge. Former resistance starts to be overcome, conflicts are patched up. A determination to complete the task is accompanied by an open exchange of views and feelings.

● Performing – the group is getting on with the task they were set up to do. Roles within the group are functional and flexible. Individuals feel safe to express differences of opinion and trust the group to find acceptable compromises. Lots of energy for group problem solving.

TEAM ORGANISATION

There are a number of practical features of team organisation which are fundamental to team success.

The purpose of the team

This should be agreed and accepted by all team members. If the purpose is clear, it is possible to clarify goals and agree priorities. By setting clear objectives, progress can be monitored. Objectives provide the basis for planning action and should be challenging but achievable, and set against a specific timescale.

The nature of the tasks or activities required to achieve team purpose will influence how the work is divided between team members.

Communication

It is important the team establishes efficient and effective methods of communication so that information can be shared; advice can be offered and sought; and consultation and negotiation can take place about ideas, plans and opinions, before decisions are made. One method is by team meetings.

Team meetings

For team meetings to be productive, planning is needed to ensure meetings are attended by well prepared members, that the purpose of the meeting is clear, it is well chaired to ensure team participation and there is accurate recording of what has taken place and what decisions have been made. This does not necessarily need to be formalised in a structure, although, for teamwork to flourish, meetings should not be left to chance. If meetings are well planned and structured, progress will be made towards achieving the team task, and members will remain motivated, enthusiastic and willing to attend. Full team meetings will not always be necessary. Smaller subgroups may be set up to respond to a very specific objective. Pritchard (1981) describes these as 'intrinsic' teams. Teams which deal with particular functions such as 'administration', 'management', 'home nursing' are known as 'functional teams'.

LEADERSHIP

If a team is to function well it must have a leader. The choice of leader will depend on several things including the make up of the team and the nature of the task the team is to perform. The team leader does not necessarily have to be the person who has the highest professional status. In any case, the leader must be truly accepted by the other team members as the leader. A team leader should:

- Have a clear vision of what he or she wants to achieve and be able to communicate it to other team members.
- Motivate other team members and be prepared to delegate.
- Recognise and harness the skills and expertise of the team members in relation to the task.
- Develop shared values and aspirations of team members.
- Head the team in a 'proactive' way.
- Be flexible, willing to listen to suggestions and adopt a range of leadership styles as appropriate to different situations.

The team leader needs to foster commitment and loyalty rather than submission and compliance. It is his or her responsibility to ensure the team works in the most efficient and effective way to achieve its goal.

STYLES OF LEADERSHIP

Democratic

This style is characterised by involving all team members in the discussion and decision making process. Providing structure and momentum to the group, he or she is prepared to mould to the needs of the group. He or she pays as much attention to how the team operates as the task the team is to perform.

The strength of this style of leadership is that it gives power to the team members, which will in time energise them to achieve the objectives.

Authoritarian

Whilst acknowledging individual team members, the authoritarian leader is not willing to give responsibility to anyone else for how the group operates. He or she is firm, definite and unbending . All power is invested in the leader. The strength of this style of leadership is that everyone is clear about their role and position within the group and tasks may be completed quickly.

The weaknesses, however, are that all members may not contribute and the team is not able to function without the presence of the leader. Team members will 'opt' out of responsibility.

Laissez-faire

This type of leader allows the team members to freely express themselves, does not seek to impose but offers suggestions which members may or may not be willing to take up. Although an important part of the group, he or she is not the final arbitrator in decisions relating to the purpose of the team or the strategies to achieve its goal. This style allows creative ideas to emerge and be explored, but can become aimless, frustrating and non-productive.

Although there is no overall 'perfect' leadership style, the democratic approach combines flexibility and involvement of all team members with some direction when required. At times though, it may be necessary to use an authoritarian style when decisions are to be made and deadlines are to be met, and a *laissez-faire* style when looking for new ideas and innovation.

MAKING DECISIONS

Most teams develop a preferred or accepted decision-making process. This can be formally agreed by the team or can be made each time a decision is required and may change according to the type of decision needed on that occasion.

Factors influencing the method chosen will include time constraints, the degree of commitment needed by team members to put the decision into action, the leadership style or power invested in team members, and the amount of 'risk' associated with the decision. Some common methods of decision making are described.

Self-authorised decisions

These are decisions taken by one member of the team without prior team consent. They are sometimes called 'executive decisions' and are usually made by a powerful high status member of the team. This method is justified in situations where an immediate response is required but, if used often, will lower commitment to team working.

Coalitions

This is where two or more team members join forces to take a decision, which other team members find difficult to oppose. This can result in the team becoming fragmented with small powerful subgroups within it. Morale of other team members is destroyed.

Majority vote

This is where the decision taken is based on the view of a majority of team members. An actual vote is not always taken. Those who 'lose the vote', however, may not be prepared to support the majority view and may even attempt to sabotage the team.

Consensus

This is where all team members are given a chance to participate in the discussion and have equal opportunity to influence the team decision. The discussion continues until all members can accept a final decision, even if it is not their preferred option. Although this method will develop team cohesion it is likely to be quite time-consuming. The team leader may therefore attempt to summarise the views of the team and make a final decision.

WHAT STEPS CAN BE TAKEN TO FACILITATE TEAMWORKING?

Understanding how teams work and taking the time to look at the workings of one's own group are among the best ways of improving team performance. This requires, however, an understanding of the benefits of working in a team and a commitment by the team members to improving the quality of their team working. It will be best to look at team processes in a particular order:

1. Goals
   - What are we here for?
   - What is the task?
2. Roles
   - Who does what?
3. Procedures
   - How do we go about it?
4. Interpersonal relationships
   - How do we get on together?

By starting at the top of the list, teams will begin to develop good interpersonal relationships and any problems can be sorted out along the way. A more comprehensive list of questions about team working follows. Working systematically through these questions with the team will help to develop a clear picture of how well the team is working, and what changes need to be made to help the team function more effectively.

QUESTIONS ABOUT TEAM WORKING (Prichard, 1981)

Aims, tasks

- Are we all here for a common purpose?
- What is that purpose?
- Do we agree about the tasks we set ourselves?
- Do we define them adequately?
- Can they be measured so that we know if the task has been completed?

Roles

- Are we clear about our own role in the team?
- Are we clear about the roles of others in the team?
- Are these roles in conflict, and if so where?
- Are we unable to fulfil our role (e.g., due to overwork)?
- Is our ability to carry out our role hampered by outside constraints (e.g., not being allowed to make decisions, fear of litigation, etc)?

Procedures

- In making decisions do we take adequate notice of:
  - who has the relevant information?
  - who has to carry out the decision?
- Are decisions usually made:
  - unanimously?
  - by majority?
  - by team leader?
  - by default?
- When a decision is made, is it carried out, or forgotten?
- Does the team follow up its decisions, question the outcome, and learn by its mistakes and successes?
- When a conflict arises do we:
  - ignore it?
  - allow one person to force a decision?
  - compromise?
  - look for alternative solutions?
- Do we let everyone have a chance to speak, or let one or two members do all the talking?
- Does everyone feel free to challenge any statements made in the group?

- Do we waste time, or allot it according to the priority of the task?
- Does the team meet often enough and in the right circumstances, and is the size of the group right?
- Do team members concentrate on the task, or waste time trying to impress, or raising irrelevant issues?

Interpersonal relationships

- Are team members sensitive to how others in the group feel about discussion?
- Can the team tolerate failure and give natural support rather than blame?
- Is team morale high? If not, why not?
- Can any member suggest any way in which team working could be improved?

Recruitment and selection

Appointing the right staff is one of the most important tasks any organisation carries out. All too often, however, interviews are badly conducted, with unbriefed interview panels, inappropriate questioning and poor general organisation. Personnel officers within FHSAs or HAs are well trained in recruitment and selection and will be available in most circumstances to help in this important process. There may be occasions, however, when you will be asked to help with the organisation and selection of new staff, either within your own department or for a general practice, for example, for a practice nurse, or to act as external assessor for some other HA.

WRITING JOB DESCRIPTIONS

The first part of the recruitment process involves identifying the key areas of responsibility and key skills required for the post. It is always difficult starting completely from scratch, so it is worth obtaining job descriptions of similar posts elsewhere.*

---

*The National Facilitator Development Project holds a selection of primary care facilitator, audit facilitator and practice nurse advisor job descriptions. The Royal College of Nursing can provide them for practice nurse posts and specimen contracts of employment.

The job description should be clear and succinct giving a brief overview of the main aims of the position, identifying who the post holder is accountable to and outlining specific areas of responsibility. It is always wise to add the proviso at the end, that the job description is not exhaustive and other duties may from time to time be necessary. This is particularly important for new posts which may develop in a slightly different way than at first expected. It is possible of course to review and rewrite the job description at an appropriate time, if the job has changed substantially.

PRE-ADVERTISING

Before you go ahead and advertise the post, make sure that the funds are available to make the appointment! Health service changes happen so quickly that funds may not be as secure as you may at first think.

You will need to know the date when funds become available and the length of the commitment. Many posts are now funded on a 'rolling' contract, which could be for two or three years. This usually means that funds are available for at least three years, but at the end of each year the employee's performance will be reviewed. If it is satisfactory then the contract will continue for another three years. If performance is not satisfactory only two years' funding will remain until reviewed again at the end of the following year. Fixed term appointments guarantee funding for a 'fixed' period, for example, one, two or three years. The post may subsequently be funded longer, but this is not guaranteed.

INTERVIEW PANEL

Arrange a short listing and date(s) for interviews with the selection panel, before the advertisement goes to press.

Selecting the appropriate interview panel is important as they will need to judge the qualities of the candidates. The interview panel should consist of: the person responsible for employing the candidate or his/her representative and the day to day 'line manager' or key liaison person. It may also include an external assessor, who can offer a very unbiased view and would hold the 'deciding vote' if that became necessary. This person may also be someone who represents the profession being interviewed for, if no other member of the panel can give that view, or have some special knowledge about the type of post on offer. Many facilitators are called on to act as external assessor when FHSAs are making new facilitator appointments.

It is always helpful to have someone from the personnel department involved in the interview if at all possible. The personnel officer can help to ensure the interviews are run fairly and do not prejudice or discriminate against any candidate.

There is no recommended number for a panel but the danger is to include too many. Make sure it includes only those who are absolutely necessary.

ADVERTISING

Picking the most appropriate journal or newspaper in order to attract the right candidate is very important. Some organisations expect the post to be advertised internally first. You can check this with the personnel department.

The advertisement should provide a brief but clear summary of the post and should state clearly the form of reply desired, for example, request for further information, letter giving past experience and qualifications or curriculum vitae. The advertisement should also give the name of the contact person for applications and a contact for informal discussion if appropriate.

Applications should be acknowledged promptly and applicants kept informed of the progress of the selection procedures. (Job description and any other information about the post should be ready for sending out immediately.)

No personal information should be requested unless relevant to the appointment and all applications should be treated as confidential.

SHORTLISTING

Assessing the applications is usually undertaken by all interviewers. The interview panel members are sent copies of all applications together with the job description and personnel specification for the post. The personnel specification is a list of the skills, experience and personal qualities the candidates will need to effectively fulfil the requirements of the post. It will be helpful at the shortlisting and interview stage. After formulating individual choices the panel usually gets together to make a final shortlisting.

The decision to interview ought to take into consideration:

- How well the candidate fulfils the requirements of the personnel specification, for example, qualifications, past experience and special skills.
- How well the job will meet the needs and aspirations of the candidate. This information may be gained from a covering

letter or short paragraph included in the application which describes why the candidate wants the post and his/her suitability.

Both of these aspects of the candidate's suitability for the post can be explored further at interview.

Reasons for not shortlisting (or appointing)

These must be clearly thought through and recorded. This information may be retained by the personnel department in case candidates subsequently enquire why. Reasons may include:

- Inappropriate or no qualifications.
- Lack of knowledge or understanding of the job.
- Incomplete or poor application.
- Late application.
- Failed selection test or medical.
- Non-attendance at interview.
- Poor references.
- Subsequent refusal of the offer.

Just not liking the applicant is not a good enough reason not to appoint, although when working closely in a small team, personalities, attitudes and beliefs will be very important.

Let the candidate know as soon as possible whether or not they are shortlisted. This is the time to request references. Make sure if candidates have asked to be consulted before references are taken up, that you do let them know *before* you do it. The candidates should also be told at this stage the date, time and expected length of interview, who to ask for when arriving and also if they will be asked, for example, to either present some of their work or give a talk on some topic of the panel's choice. It will also be helpful if you clarify whether flipcharts, overhead projectors or other equipment will be made available.

THE INTERVIEW

Preparation

Good interviews require thorough preparation by the interviewer as well as the interviewees.

General organisation

Book rooms for the interview and waiting area as soon as possible and ensure there is the space for presentation equipment if this is necessary. On the day, one member of the staff should be responsible for receiving the candidates and bringing them to the interview room when appropriate. The room should be roomy but not too large and unfriendly. Comfortable semi-formal seating is best arranged in a circle or semi-circle facing the candidate.

If possible, the use of a desk behind which the panel sits should be avoided but a low coffee table can provide a place for papers and drinks if necessary.

The room should be a comfortable temperature and in a quiet part of the building. If telephones cannot be removed, all calls should be diverted elsewhere.

The panel should be aware of the interview timing and have copies of all applications, a job description, the candidate's references (usually only referred to at the very end of the interview) and any scoring forms, etc., that are to be used.

The objectives of the interview

The interview is intended to:

- Provide the panel with an opportunity to ascertain the candidate's suitability for the post and give the candidate a fair hearing.
- Provide the candidate with an opportunity to assess the job and the organisation, and to demonstrate his or her suitability to the post.

It is, therefore, important to clarify the subject areas for questioning, plan the questions and allocate them to the suitable interviewer and prepare for the candidate's questions. The interview is not designed to 'trip up' the candidate and the panel should therefore work hard to ensure the candidate feels as comfortable and relaxed as possible.

The format of the interview

The chairperson of the interview panel welcomes the candidate, offers a seat, and introduces the other panel members and their subject area for questioning. The chairperson can then begin the questioning in areas in which the candidate is familiar such as their present job, their interest in this post, etc.

Encouraging the candidate to speak freely means using open questions such as 'Tell us about . . .', 'What is your opinion of . . .'. Closed questions can be used for points of clarification and general information.

The questioning usually passes to each interviewer in turn and may finish with the chairperson picking up any further points not already covered. The chairperson can, however, give the interviewers the opportunity to ask any further questions and it is helpful to negotiate this with the chair first.

The candidate is then given an opportunity to ask questions before the chairperson clarifies practical points such as length of notice required, contact telephone number, etc. You may also like to ask if the candidate, in the light of the interview, is still interested in the post.

The candidate is then thanked for attending and told when the results of the interview will be made known to them. They should also be given an expenses form to complete and give to the reception person before leaving.

It is acceptable and indeed desirable to make notes during the interview and to spend a few minutes at the end of each summarising your impressions. It is usual to leave any discussion about the candidates until all the interviews have been carried out.

Using a presentation

Many organisations expect candidates to make a presentation of their views on some aspect of the post on offer. The title may be given to the candidates when they are invited to interview, or can be given as the candidate arrives. They should be informed of this aspect of the selection process beforehand, however, and asked to arrive 30 minutes early in order to prepare their talk. This is usually only expected to last for about 10 minutes.

This method does give the candidate an opportunity to put over his or her views and discuss the issues he or she is familiar with. The main advantage for the interviewer is to get a better picture of the breadth and depth of knowledge the candidate has and to see how well the candidate 'performs' when presenting. If this is not likely to be part of the job, however, the content rather than the presentation skills should be the focus of attention.

The presentation should also demonstrate other aspects of the candidate's views, attitudes and non-verbal as well as verbal communication style, which would not normally come through in the usual question and answer interview style.

The presentation is usually done after the first introductory part of the interview and before the questions proper begin.

Selecting the candidate

At the end of all the interviews each panel member should complete and summarize any notes that have been taken during the interviews.

There is no hard and fast rule about who has their say first. Sometimes the external assessor is asked to begin and at other times they are asked to give their opinions last of all. Each panel member should give a summary of the strengths and weaknesses of each candidate in relation to the job specification before excluding any candidates who are deemed 'not appointable'. Tentative ratings on suitability should be made by each panel member before confirming with others. Judgements should be rational and based on the information gathered at the interview and should not be influenced by bias, irrelevances and prejudices.

Only consensus decision is acceptable and if this cannot be reached it may be wise to either call some candidates back for second interview or to re-advertise and start the process again. It is never advisable to appoint a candidate if there is any doubt about his or her ability to do the job well.

AFTER THE SELECTION PROCESS

All application forms, CVs, etc., are collected by personnel for disposal. Candidates should be promptly informed of the decision. The successful candidate is usually contacted by telephone and followed by a letter of confirmation. Unsuccessful candidates may also be telephoned, if this has been previously agreed. In any case, each candidate is sent a letter to confirm the panel's decision.

SOME FINAL WORDS OF WARNING

There are a number of factors that can bias or distort the rational assessment of candidates.

The 'halo' effect

When assessing a candidate it is important to beware of the 'halo' effect. This means giving a candidate either high or low ratings in all aspects of the job specification because of one striking characteristic, for example, an exceptional event in which a candidate was involved, having something in common with an interviewer, or having made a wrong choice or mistake during their past career.

Contrast with other interviewees

Candidates should be assessed on their own merits and although difficult not to do, comparison with other candidates is inappropriate in anything other than the specifications for the post.

Stereotyping

This can cause an inability to recognise the relevant qualities of the candidate.

Level of accuracy of recall

If inconclusive notes are made on the candidates at the time of interview, the interviewer may find it difficult to recall the characteristics of all the candidates. It is very important, therefore, to make adequate notes.

Discrimination

It is most important that recruitment and selection of new employees is fair to all applicants and potential applicants and does not in effect discriminate against minority groups, members of one sex or marital status. Disabled candidates may also be unwittingly discriminated against, even when the disability will not adversely affect their performance in that job. It is feasible of course to discuss any adjustments needed to allow the applicant to do the job but the decision to appoint should always be based on the ability to do the job, irrespective of the disability.

Time management

WHAT DO WE MEAN BY TIME MANAGEMENT?

Managing your time effectively does not mean being 'busy' every minute of the day. It does imply, however, spending some time thinking about how you use your time to make the most of the time you have available. It involves planning and prioritising activities, while remaining flexible to deal with urgent or unforeseen events.

Whenever we undertake a task, we make a decision, whether consciously or unconsciously, to do that particular thing at that moment instead of doing something else. A general principle of good time-management is to ensure that, as far as possible in those areas of working life that you are able to control, decision-making is a conscious process.

HOW WELL DO YOU MANAGE YOUR TIME?

Before going on to look at time management in detail, complete the following questionnaire to see how well you are doing. (This has been adapted from Steel, 1986; original source: Brunel University Time Management Course).

Below are 10 statements that suggest good time management. Answer these items by putting a tick next to the item most characteristic of how you carry out your job. Use the information on page 124 to check your answers and find your score.

1. *Each day I set aside a small amount of time for planning and thinking about my job.*
   - Almost never
   - Sometimes
   - Often
   - Almost always

2. *I set specific, written goals and put deadlines on them.*
   - Almost never
   - Sometimes
   - Often
   - Almost always

3. *I make a daily 'to do' list, arrange items in order of importance, and try to get the important items done as soon as possible.*
   - Almost never
   - Sometimes
   - Often
   - Almost always

4. *I am aware of the 80–20 rule and use it in doing my job.* (The 80–20 rule states that 80 per cent of your effectiveness will generally come from achieving only 20 per cent of your goals.)
   - Almost never
   - Sometimes
   - Often
   - Almost always

5. *I keep a loose schedule to allow for crises and the unexpected.*
   - Almost never
   - Sometimes
   - Often
   - Almost always

6. *I delegate everything I can to others.*
   - Almost never
   - Sometimes
   - Often
   - Almost always

7. *I try to handle each piece of paper only once.*
   - Almost never
   - Sometimes
   - Often
   - Almost always

8. *I eat a light lunch so I don't get sleepy in the afternoon.*
   - Almost never
   - Sometimes
   - Often
   - Almost always

9. *I make an active effort to keep common interruptions (visitors, meetings, telephone calls) from continually disrupting my working day.*
   - Almost never
   - Sometimes
   - Often
   - Almost always

10. *I am able to say no to others' requests for my time if this would prevent my completing important tasks.*
    - Almost never
    - Sometimes
    - Often
    - Almost always

To get your score, give yourself:
   3 points for each 'Almost always'
   2 points for each 'Often'
   1 point for each 'Sometimes'
   0 points for each 'Almost never'

Add up your points to get your total score

If you scored:

   0–15   Better give some thought to managing your time.
   15–20   You're doing OK but there's room for improvement.
   20–25   Very good.
   25–27   Excellent.
   28–30   You cheated!

It may be helpful to reflect for a moment on how you spend your day. List the sorts of activities you are involved in and draw a pie chart to represent the amount of time spent on each. It may look something like Fig. 6.3.

In this way, you will be able to see which activities take up most of your time. Is this the way you would like to use your time, or is there a more effective way? In fact, what tends to happen, is that we stretch the working day and allow it to eat into our leisure or family time instead of really tackling the way we organise our working day.

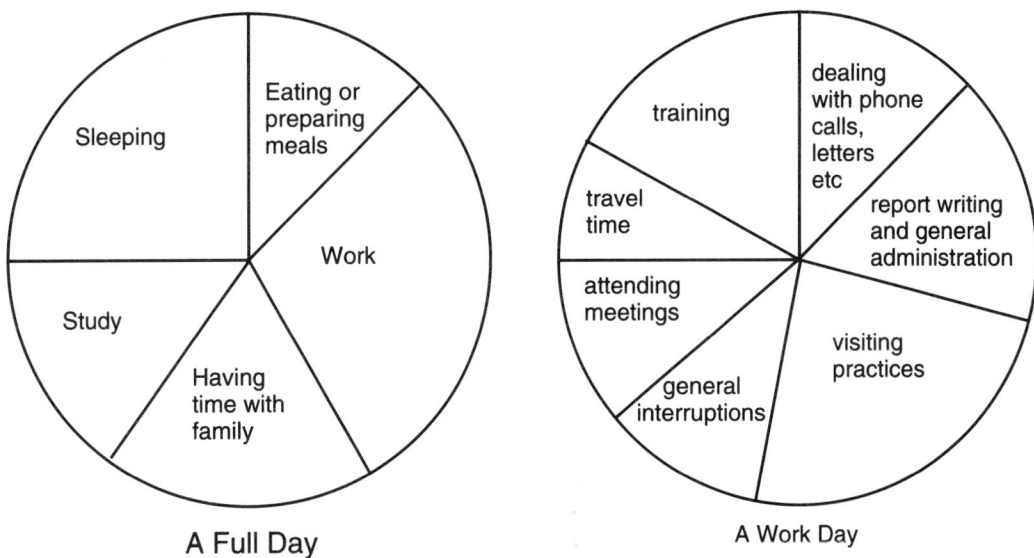

Figure 6.3. Pie charts representing amount of time spent on activities

PLANNING DAY-TO-DAY WORK

'Planning is bringing the future into the present so that you can do something about it now!' (Alan Lakein, 1984.)

Some might think that planning work is a waste of time – you could be doing the work instead! Writers on time management argue that proper planning is a good investment and, in any case, it need not take up that much time – 10 minutes per day plus a half-hour review session at the end of the week is probably adequate.

The time management routine offered below has been shown to be useful. However, time management does involve considerable self-discipline and there may be times when you are unable to apply the system as conscientiously as you would like.

Make a 'TO DO' list

Include all the long-, medium- and short-term projects and activities you are involved with, both large and small scale.

Set priorities

The activities in your day can probably be classed according to urgency or importance. You may find it helpful to use the grid in Fig. 6.4.

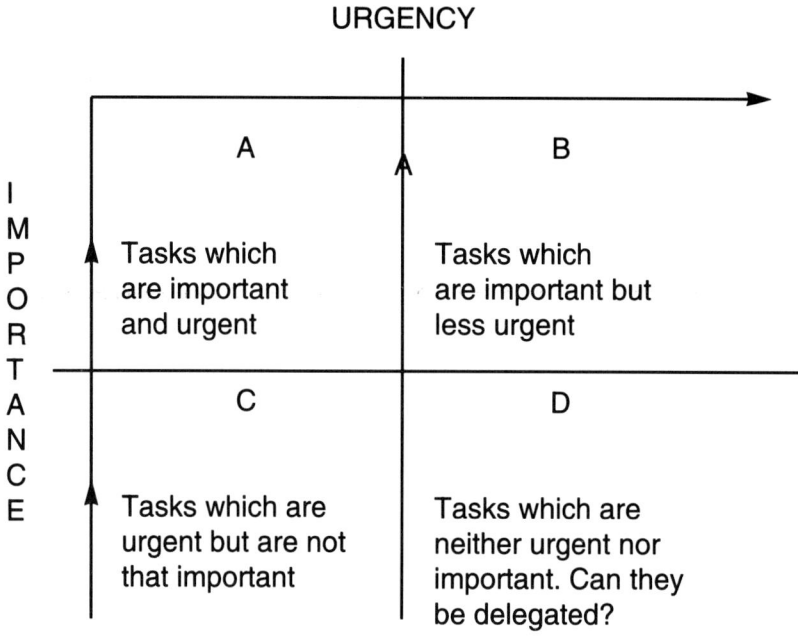

Figure 6.4. Suggested grid for dividing up daily activities

Tasks of:

- High priority, A, are important and urgent.
- Medium priority, B, are either important but not urgent or urgent but not important.
- Low priority, C, are neither urgent nor important and you should consider either not doing them or delegating them to someone else.

You may also need to break each of these groups down further according to the urgency with which each has to be completed – A1, A2, A3, B1, B2, etc.

There is no right or wrong way to list priorities, it is largely a matter of guesswork and intuition – the As, Bs and Cs will change over time or due to unforeseen circumstances. The As usually stand out clearly, Bs and Cs are more difficult.

Produce a work schedule

Decide exactly what you will do when, taking note of your list of priorities:

- Weekly
  - Block out (by putting a line through the relevant time in your

diary) previously determined commitments, for example, meetings. (These can also be prioritised – listed or coded in terms of priority.)
   – Block out times for completing category A tasks.
   – Use any time left to block out any B or C tasks.

● You could also block out set times each day (say in the morning) for routine items, for example, paperwork or filing and/or longer blocks of time (say one afternoon per week) to work on longer on-going projects. The success of this stage depends on being able to estimate how long tasks will take.
● Daily
   – Go through your plan and add any new items that need to be included.
   – List the tasks you have to complete that day using the ABC priority system.
   – Any As that do not get done should go on the list for the next day.

Review of the week's work

At a convenient point in the week – usually Friday or Monday – look closely at your lists and check how far down the As, Bs and Cs you have got. This will form the basis of the next week's plan. Bs and Cs which you have not done may now be urgent enough to have an A priority.

If you feel you and/or your work would benefit from developing your time-management skills try using this system to plan your work over the next few weeks. Non-work time can also be included in a planning routine – a particularly useful ploy if and when you find work spilling over into leisure time. You may be able to devise a routine of your own or adapt this one to make it more relevant to your needs. Take some time to experiment with ideas until you find what works best for you.

DEALING WITH PAPERWORK

Aim to handle each piece of paper (e.g. letters) only once. Do whatever you can straight away so you do not have to waste time re-reading items and thinking yourself back into the task.

Develop a classification system for sorting piles of paper. For example, you could mark papers:

● Action, for immediate attention, for example, routine letters, telephone calls, matters which can be delegated.
● Information, to read and digest later, for example, complex

letters, minutes of meetings, reports, information, for filing.
● Deferred, keep for spare moments, for example, papers, journals, non-urgent reports.

You will also save time and duplication of effort by writing notes for answering letters and instructions for filing and follow-up directly onto the papers.

COPING WITH INFORMATION OVERLOAD

Reading journals, books, periodicals, reports, etc. to keep up with developments in your field of work can seem like a full-time job in itself. You could ease the burden in one or more of the following ways.

● Make reading part of your work routine. Try to set aside a period of time (say 30 minutes) at the same time each day (perhaps immediately before lunch or before leaving work in the evening).
● Spend some time reading as a means of relaxing. This is especially useful after you have done a stint of really concentrated activity, for example, writing a report, attending a meeting.
● Develop your ability to skim-read. Just make a few notes on a card index file for future reference.
● Make a habit of skimming through one book or weighty article each day. This will at least ensure you are making some impression on the mass of materials coming your way.

IDENTIFY PRIME TIMES

There are two sorts of prime time:

● Internal, the time of day when you are able to work best. This is the time to use for working on complex creative tasks.
● External, times in the day when other people are likely to be around, for example, to give information, make decisions or attend meetings.

You can save a lot of time and frustration by checking out what the prime times of your main professional client groups are. Doctors can often only be contacted at each end of the working day or after morning surgery. People are often willing to use the 12–2 p.m. period to attend a meeting that includes a working lunch.

Your work schedules will be more effective if you utilise your's and other people's prime times.

CREATING QUIET/THINKING TIMES

Blocking out times for working on complex tasks does not guarantee you will be left alone to get on with them. Some of the following strategies might help:

- Let others around you know when you do not want to be disturbed, for example, by visitors or phone calls.
- Try to find a quiet room or library to work in.
- Ask for advance warning of complex tasks so you have time to put them into your work schedule. When, as inevitably happens, something is dropped on you unexpectedly, establish what sort of priority it should have over things with which you are already dealing.

COPING WITH OTHER PEOPLE'S DEMANDS

Meeting other people's demands will have to be prioritised within your work schedule along with your other commitments. The following points are worth considering.

- Saying 'yes' and not coming up with the goods is often worse than saying 'no' (with a reasonable explanation) in the first place. Saying 'no' does at least give the person concerned the opportunity to explore other options and/or make other arrangements.
- If someone demands something quickly, they are probably looking for speed rather than perfection – accept the fact that you usually cannot achieve both.
- Look for ways of redirecting or delegating demands you cannot meet – you may be able to spend a little time offering helpful suggestions even if you cannot carry out the task yourself.
- If demands become too much to cope with, you may need to review your workload, work methods and priorities.
- Consider the costs involved when you decide to change your plans to meet a new demand. The activity not only has a cost in terms of your salary, overheads, etc., it also has a cost in terms of the benefits forgone. You therefore need to decide which of the options is of most value.

(Adapted from the HEO Training Manual; Steel, 1986)

7 Additional information

Useful journals

British Medical Journal, PO Box 295, London, WC1H 9TE. Tel: 071-387-4499.

Health Education Journal, Distribution Section, Health Education Authority, Hamilton House, Mabeldon Place, London, WC1H 9TX. Tel: 071-383-3833.

Health Education Research, Journal Subscriptions Department, Oxford University Press, Walton Street, Oxford, OX2 6DP. Tel: 0865 56767.

Health Services Journal, Macmillan Magazines Ltd, 4 Little Essex Street, London, WX2R 3LF. Tel: 071-240-1101.

Health Trends, HMSO Publications Centre, PO Box 276, London, SW8 5DT. Tel: 071-873-0011.

Health Visitors Journal, BMA House, Tavistock Square, London, WC1H 9LR. Tel: 071-383-6243.

International Journal of Health Care Quality Assurance, MCB University Press Ltd, 60–62 Toller Lane, Bradford. Tel: 0274 499821.

Journal of the Royal College of General Practitioners, 14 Princes Gate, Hyde Park, London, SW7 1PU. Tel: 071-581-3232.

Network Magazine, Medical Audit Association, Room G, Cleethorpes Centre, Jackson Place, Wilton Road, Humberston, S. Humberside. Tel: 0472 210687.

Nursing Standard, Viking House, 17–19 Peterborough Road, Harrow, Middlesex, HA1 2AX. Tel: 071-423-1066.

Nursing Times, Macmillan Magazines Ltd, 4 Little Essex Street, London, WC2 3LF. Tel: 071-240-1101.

Practical Diabetes (Incorporating *Diabetes in General Practice*

Supplement), The Newbourne Group, Maxwell Consumer Publishing & Communications Ltd, Greater London House, Hampstead Road, Freepost, London, NW1 3YP. Tel: 071-383-3444.

Practice Nurse, Reed Healthcare Communications Ltd, Friary Court, 13-21 High Street, Guildford, GU1 3DX. Tel: 0483-502125.

Practice Nursing, Mark Allen Group Publications, Croxted Mews, 288 Croxted Road, London, SE24 9DA. Tel: 081-6717521.

Primary Health Care, The Journal for Community Health Nurses, BMJ Publishing Group, BMA House, Tavistock Square, London, WC1H 9JR. Tel: 081 423 1066.

Quality Assurance in Health Care, BMJ Publishing Group, BMA House, Tavistock Square, London, WC1H 9JR. Tel: 071-383-6339.

Bibliography

Ackerman, W. B. & Lohnes, P. R. (1981). *Research Methods for Nurses*. McGraw-Hill Book Company, Maidenhead.

Act Pack (1991). *Teamwork in Practice*. Radcliffe Medical Press Ltd, Oxford.

Adair, J. (1986). *Effective Teambuilding*. Gower, London.

Allsop, J. (1984). *Health Policy and the National Health Service*. Longman Group UK Ltd, Harlow.

Allsop, J. (1990). *Changing Primary Care: The Role of Facilitator*. Kings Fund Centre Primary Health Care Group, London.

Argyle, M. (1973). *Social Interaction*, Tavistock Publications, London.

Armstrong, D., Calnan, M. & Grace, J. (1990). *Research Methods for General Practitioners*. Oxford University Press, Oxford.

Baker, R. & Priestly, P. (1990). *The Practice Audit Plan*. Severn Faculty Royal College of General Practitioners, Bristol.

Belbin, R. M. (1981). *Management Teams: Why They Succeed or Fail*. Heineman, London.

Bond, T. (1986). *Games for Social and Life Skills*. Hutchinson, London.

Butcher, J. (1992). *Copy Editing. The Cambridge Handbook for Editors, Authors and Publishers*. Cambridge University Press, Cambridge.

Chisholm, J. (Ed.) (1990). *Making Sense of the New Contract*. Radcliffe Medical Press Ltd, Oxford.

Cockburn, J., Ruth, D., Silagy, C. *et al.* (1991). Randomised trial of three approaches for marketing smoking cessation programmes to Australia general practitioners. *British Medical Journal*, **304**, 691–4.

Collins, J. (1983). *Activities and Ideas. Handbook of Games for Communication Groups*. Winslow Press, Bicester.

Coronary Prevention Group (1990). *Coronation Heart Disease Statistics Factsheet*. Coronary Prevention Group, London.

Danow, S. & Bailey, C. (1990). *Developing Skills with People*. Wiley, Chichester.

Dietrich, A. J., O'Conner, G. T., Keiler, A., Carney, P. A., Levy, D. & Whaley, F. S. (1992). Cancer: improving early detection and prevention. A community practice randomised trial. *British Medical Journal*, **304**, 687–91.

Department of Health (1989a). Health Circular (FP) (89) 20.

Department of Health (1989b). *General Practice in the NHS: The 1990 Contract*. HMSO, London.

Department of Health (1990a). *Medical Audit in the Family Practitioners Services*. HMSO, London.

Department of Health (1990b). *NHS General Medical Services Statement of Fees and Allowances Payable to General Medical Practitioners in England and Wales*. HMSO, London.

Department of Health (1992a). *The Patient's Charter*. (HPC1). HMSO, London.

Department of Health (1992b). *The Health of the Nation*. (CM 1986). HMSO, London.

Department of Health (1993a). *The Health of the Nation*. Key Area Handbooks. HMSO, London.

Department of Health (1993b). *Audit Guidelines for Health Promotion Banding*. HMSO, London.

Department of Health and Social Security (1965). *Charter for the Family Doctor Service*. HMSO, London.

Department of Health and Social Security (1983). *NHS Management Enquiry Report*. The Griffiths Report. HMSO, London.

Donabedian, A. (1980a). Exploration in quality assessment and monitoring. In *Human Service Quality. An Introduction to Quality Methods for Health Services*, ed. J. Øvretveit (1992). Blackwell, Oxford.

Donabedian, A. (1980b). *The Definition of Quality and Approaches to its Assessment*, vol. 1. Health Administration Press, Michigan.

Donabedian, A. (1988). Quality assessment and assurance unity of purpose, diversity of means. *Inquiry*, **25**, 173–92.

Ewles, L. & Simnet, I. (1992). *Promoting Health* – A Practical Guide to Health Education. John Wiley & Sons Ltd., Chichester.

Fender, H. (1991). Facilitators in Primary Health Care. M. Med. Sci. Dissertation.

Field, J. & Henderson J. (1992). *Better Living Better Life*. Knowledge House Ltd, Henley on Thames.

Fullard, E., Fowler, G. & Gray, M. (1987). Promoting prevention in primary care: controlled trial of low technology. Low cost approach. *British Medical Journal*, **294**, 1080–2.

Gilmore, M., Bruce, N. & Hunt, M. (1974). *The Work of the Nursing Team in General Practice*. Central Council for Education and Training for Health Visitors, London.

Ham, C. (1991). *The New National Health Service Organisation and Management*. Radcliffe Medical Press, Oxford.

Hayes, J. (1991). *Interpersonal Skills. Goal Directed Behaviour at Work*. Harper Collins Academic, London.

Hughes, S. & Humphries, C. (1990). *Medical Audit in General Practice. A practical guide to the literature*. Kings Fund Centre, London.

International Journal of Health Care Quality Assurance – source of useful articles, *see* 'Useful journals'.

Irvine, D. & Irvine, S. (Eds) (1991). *Making Sense of Audit*. Radcliffe Medical Press, Oxford.

Kanter, R. M. (1983). *The Change Masters*. Unwin Hyman Ltd, London.

Lakein, A. (1984). *How to Get Control of Your Time and Your Life*. Gower, Aldershot.

Marinker, M. (Ed.) (1990). *Medical Audit & General Practice*. British Medical Foundation, London.

Maxwell, R. J. (1984). Perspective in NHS management. Quality assessment in health. *British Medical Journal*, **288**, 1470–2.

National Facilitator Development Project (1992). *Strategy Review*. (Unpublished. Available from National Facilitator Development Project.)

Neighbour, R. (1987). *The Inner Consultation. How to Develop an Effective and Instructive Consulting Style*. MTP Press Ltd, Lancaster.

Network Magazine (Medical Audit Association) – source of useful information, *see* 'Useful journals'.

Office of Population Census and Surveys (OPCS) *Mortality Statistics*. Available from HMSO bookshops.

Office of Public Service and Science (1991). *The Citizen's Charter*. (CM 1599). HMSO, London.

Øvretveit, J. (Ed.) (1992). *Health Service Quality: An Introduction to Quality Methods for Health Services*. Blackwell, Oxford.

Peters, T. (1988). *Thriving on Chaos*. Macmillan Ltd. London.

Peters, T. & Austin, N. (1985). *A Passion for Excellence*. Collins, London.

Pringle, M., Bilhhu, J., Dornan, M. & Head, S. (1991). *Managing Change in Primary Care*. Radcliffe Medical Press, Oxford.

Pritchard, P. (1981) *Manual of Primary Health Care*. (2nd edn.) Oxford University Press, Oxford.

Royal College of General Practitioners (1981). *Prevention of Arterial Disease in General Practice* No. 19. Royal College of General Practitioners, London.

Sage, G. (1991). Customers and the NHS. *International Journal of Health Care Quality Assurance*, **4**(3), 11–14.

Secretary of State for Health (1989a). *Caring for People*. (Cmn 849). HMSO, London.

Secretary of State for Health (1989b). *Working for Patients*. (Cmn 555). HMSO, London.

Secretary of State for Social Services (1987). *Promoting Better Health*. (Cmn 249). HMSO, London.

Shaper, A. G. (1988). *CHD Risks and Reasons*. Current Medical Literature Ltd, London.

Shaper, A. G., Pocock, S. J., Walker,. M., Cohen, N. M., Wale, C. J. & Thomson, A. G. (1982). British Regional Heart Study: cardiovascular risk factors in middle-aged men in 24 towns. *British Medical Journal*, **283**: 179–86.

Sheldon, T. A., Song, F., Davy Smith, G., Freemantle, N., Hason, J. & Long, A. (1993). *Effective Health Care*, No. 6. University of Leeds, Leeds.

Speigel, N., Murphy, E., Kinmonth, A., Ross, F., Bain J. & Coates, R. (1992). Managing change in general practice: a step by step guide. *British Medical Journal*, **304**, 231–4.

Spurgeon, P. (Ed.) (1990). *The Changing Face of the National Health Service in the 1990s*. Longman, Harlow.

Steel, S. (1986). *Working in Health Education a Practical Manual for the Initial Training of Health Education Officers*. National Exchange College, Cambridge.

The Learning Delivery System (1991). *Focus on the Face to Face: Interpersonal Communication*. Lifeskills Communication Ltd, Leeds.

Totten, C. (ed.) (1992). *Developing Quality in Health Education and Health Promotion*. Society of Health Education and Health Promotion Specialists, Lisburn.

Townsend, P. & Davidson, N. (Eds) (1982). *Inequalities in Health – The Black Report*. Penguin Books, Harmondsworth.

Turrill, T. (1986). *Change and Innovation. A Challenge for the NHS*. Institute of Health and Management, London.

Wilson, J. M. G. & Junger, H. (1968). *Principles and Practices in Screening for Disease*. WHO, Geneva.

Resources and further reading

These are listed by subject.

ALCOHOL

Cutting Down Your Drinking *A Guide for Health Professionals* (Training Pack)	Health Education Authority Hamilton House, Mabledon Place, London WC1H 9TX.
Alcohol and Health *A Handbook for Nurses,* *Midwives* *and Health Visitors*	Catherine Hartz, Moria Plant and Malcolm Watts (1990) Medical Council on Alcoholism 1 St Andrews Place, London NW1 4LB.
Alcohol Problems *Practical Guides for General* *Practice No. 5*	Peter Anderson, Paul Wallace and Heather Jones (1988) Oxford Medical Publications, Oxford University Press, Walton Street, Oxford OX2 6DP.
Alcohol Education *A Handbook for Health and* *Welfare Professionals*	Barbara Howe (1989) Tavistock/Routledge
Better Living, Better Life	J. Field and J. Henderson (1992) Knowledge House Ltd., Henley on Thames.

AUDIT

Making Sense of Audit	Donald and Sally Irvine (May 1991) Radcliffe Medical Press Ltd, 15 Kings Meadow, Ferry Hinksey Road Oxford OX2 0DP.
Medical Audit in General Practice *A Practical Guide to the* *Literature*	Jane Hughes and Charlotte Humphrey (1990) Kings Fund Centre, 126 Albert Street, London NW1 7NF.

Guidelines for Audit in General Practice (Not published; rewritten 1993)	Available from: Elaine Fullard National Facilitator Development Project, HEA Primary Health Care Unit, The Churchill Hospital, Headington, Oxford OX3 7LJ.
Medical Audit and General Practice	Edited by Marshall Marinker (1990) The British Medical Foundation, Tavistock Square, London WC1H 9JR.
The Practice Audit Plan	R. Baker and P. Priestly (1990) Severn Faculty, RCGP Bristol.
Working for Patients	HMSO, London (1989)
Audit Guidelines for Health Promotion Banding	Department of Health (1993) (Available from FHSAs.)

BLOOD PRESSURE AND HYPERTENSION

ABC of Hypertension	A collection of articles from the *British Medical Journal*. Published 1985 by BMA, Tavistock Square, London WC1H 9JR
Hypertension	J. Tudor Hart (1987) Library of General Practice, Churchill Livingstone Medical Division of the Longman Group Ltd.

CERVICAL SCREENING

Cervical Screening – A Practical Guide	Ann McPherson (1992) Oxford Medical Publications, Oxford University Press, Published under the auspices of the Royal College of General Practitioners and the Imperial Cancer Research Fund.

CHILD HEALTH/IMMUNISATION

Immunizing Children	Sue Sefi and Aidan Macfarlane (1992) Oxford Medical publications, Oxford University Press, Walton Street, Oxford OX2 6DP.
Child Health – The Screening Tests	Aidan Macfarlane, Sue Sefi and Mario Cordeiro (1989) Oxford Medical Publications, Oxford University Press, Walton Street, Oxford OX2 6DP.
Protect Your Child with the New HIB Immunization. The Safest Way to Protect Your Child	A joint initiative of the Health Education Authority and the Department of Health (1992) Health Education Authority, Hamilton House, Mabledon Place, London WC1H 9TX

COMMUNICATION SKILLS

Working one to one	Martin Evans and Alyson Learmonth (1990) A Vital Communication, 69 Derwent Close, Cambridge CB1 4DY.
The Consultation An Approach to Learning and Teaching	David Pendleton, Theo Schofield, Peter Tate & Peter Havelock (1984) Oxford Medical Publications, Oxford University Press, Walton Street, Oxford OX2 6DP.
Developing Skills with People Training for Persons to Person Client Contact	Sheila Dainow and Caroline Bailey (1990) John Wiley & Sons Ltd, Baffins Lane, Chichester PO19 1UD.

Social Interaction	Michael Argyle (1973) Tavistock Publishers, ITPS, Chariton House, Northway, Andover, Hampshire SP10 5BE.
Games for Social and Life Skills	T. Bond (1986) Hutchinson Publishers, 62–65 Chandos Place, London WC2N 4NW.
Activities and Ideas Handbook of Games for Communication Groups	J. Collins (1986) Winslow Press, Telford Road, Bicester, Oxon OX6 7TS.
Interpersonal Skills Goal Directed Behaviour at Work	J. Hayes (1991) Harper Collins Academic, Wester Hill Road, Bishopsbriggs, Glasgow G64 2QT.
Focus on the Face to Face Interpersonal Communication	The Learning Delivery System (1991) Lifeskills Communication Ltd, Warfebank House, Ilkley Road, Otley, W. Yorks LS21 3JP.
The Inner Consultation How to Develop an Effective and Instructive Consultation Style	R. Neighbour (1987) MTP Press Ltd., Falcon House, Lancaster.

CORONARY HEART DISEASE

Lipids and Heart Disease A Practical Approach	Mann and Ball (1990) Oxford University Press, Walton Street, Oxford OX2 6DP.
CHD Risks and Reasons	A. G. Shaper (1988) Current Medical Literature Ltd, 40–42 Oshaburgh St., London NW1 3ND.
The Health of the Nation A Strategy for Health in England	Department of Health (1992) (CM 1986) HMSO, London.

The Health of the Nation Key Area Handbooks. CHD and Stroke	Department of Health (1993) HMSO, London. Available from: BAPS Health Publications Unit, Heywood Stores, No 2 Site, Manchester Road, Heywood, Lancashire OL10 2PZ.
Proposals for Nutritional Guidelines for Health Education in Britain NACNE Report	HEC, now HEA (1983)
Proposals for nutritional Diet and Cardiovascular Disease COMA Report	*Department of Health and Social Security (1984) HMSO, London.*
Does Stress Cause Heart Attacks? Psychosocial Factors in CHD	The Coronary Prevention Group (1985) Plantation House, 31–35 Fenchurch Street, London EC3M 3NN.
An Action Plan for Preventing Coronary Heart Disease in Primary Care	The Coronary Prevention Group (1991) Plantation House, 31–35 Fenchurch Street, London EC3M 3NN.
Better Living, Better Life	J. Field and J. Henderson (1992) Knowledge House Ltd., Henley on Thames.
Coronary Prevention Group	Coronary Heart Disease Statistics Factsheet (1990) The Coronary Prevention Group, Plantation House, 31–35 Fenchurch Street, London EC3M 3NN.

DIABETES

Diabetes
A Guide to Patient Management
for Practice Nurses

Jennifer Farr and Maggie
Watkinson
Radcliffe Medical Press Ltd,
15 King's Meadow, Ferry
Hinksey Road, Oxford OX2
0DP.

The Diabetics' Diet Book
A New High Fibre Eating
Programme

Dr Jim Mann and the Oxford
Dietetic Group
Martin Dunitz Ltd.

Diabetes in Practice

Henry Connor and Andrew J.
M. Bolton (1989)
John Wiley & Sons, Baffins
Lane, Chichester PO19 1UD

ABC of Diabetes

Peter J. Watkins (1993)
A collection of articles from
the *British Medical Journal*,
Published by BMA, Tavistock
Square, London WC1H 9JR.

THE ELDERLY

Preventive Care of the Elderly:
A Literature Review for the
Development of Policy and
Practice

Elizabeth Perkins (1989)
Nottingham Health Promotion
Community Unit, Memorial
House, Standard Hill,
Nottingham NG1 6FX.

Health Checks for the Over 75s
Working within the 1990 Contract

Edited by Elizabeth Perkins
(1990)
Nottingham Health Promotion
Community Unit, Memorial
House, Standard Hill,
Nottingham NG1 6FX.

EPIDEMIOLOGY

Epidemiology for the Uninitiated	G. Rose and D. J. P. Barker (1986) *British Medical Journal* Tavistock Square, London WC1H 9JR.
Epidemiology in General Practice	D. Morrell (Ed.) (1988) Oxford University Press, Walton Street, Oxford OX2 6DP.
Inequalities in Health – The Black Report	P. Townsend and N. Davidson (Eds), (1982) Penguin Books, Harmondsworth.
The Health Divide – Inequalities in Health in the 1980s	M. Whitehead (1987), HEC now HEA, London.
Mapping the Epidemic (CHD)	Health Education Authority (1990) Hamilton House, Mabledon Place, London WC1H 9TX.
Essential Community Medicine	R. J. Donaldson and L. J. Donaldson (1987) MTP Press Ltd, Falcon House, Lancaster.

FACILITATION AND PRIMARY HEALTH CARE

Manual of Primary Health Care	P. Pritchard (1981) Oxford University Press, Oxford.
General Practice in the NHS: The 1990 Contract	Department of Health (1989) HMSO, London.
Promoting prevention in primary care: controlled trial of low technology, lost cost approach.	E. Fullard, G. Fowler and M. Gray (1987) *British Medical Journal*, **294**: 1080–82.

Cancer: improving early detection and prevention. A community practice randomised trial.	A. J. Deitrich, G. T. O'Conner, A. Keiler, P. A. Carney and F. S. Waley (1992) *British Medical Journal*, **304**: 687–92.
Changing Primary Care: The Role of Facilitators	Judith Allsop (1990) Kings Fund Centre, 126 Albert Street, London NW1 7NF.
Making Sense of the New Contract	J. Chisholme (Ed.) (1990) Radcliffe Medical Press, 15 King's Meadow, Ferry Hinskey Road Oxford OX2 0DP.
Primary Health Care Team Workshop Manual A Guide to Planning and Managing Workshops for Primary Health Care Teams	Health Education Authority (1992) Hamilton House, Mabledon Place, London WC1H 9TX.

HEALTH EDUCATION/PUBLIC HEALTH

Helping People Change Risk Management Training Manual	Health Education Authority (1993) Hamilton House, Mabledon Place, London WC1H 9TX.
Promoting Health – A Practical Guide to Health Education	Linda Ewles and Ina Simnett (1992) John Wiley & Sons Ltd., Baffins Lane, Chichester PO19 1UD.
Health Promotion, Models and Values	R. S. Downie, Carol Fyfe and Andrew Tannahill (1990) Oxford University Press, Walton Street, Oxford OX2 6DP.
Disease Prevention and Health Promotion in Primary Health Care. Evaluation Report	Jill Spratley (1989) Health Education Authority, Hamilton House, Mabledon Place, London WC1H 9TX.

The Nation's Health – A Strategy for the 1990s	Alwin Smith and Bobby Jacobson (Eds.) (1980) Kings Fund Centre, 126 Albert Street, London NW1 7NF.
Health Education Perspectives and Choices	Ian Sutherland (1987) National Extension College Trust, Brooklands Avenue, Cambridge.

MANAGING CHANGE

Change and Innovation A Challenge for the NHS	Tony Turrell (1986) Institute of Health Services Management, 75 Portland Place, London W1N 4MN
A Passion for Excellence	T. Peters and N. Austin (1985) Collins, 77–78 Fulham Palace Road, London W6 8JB.
Thriving on Chaos	T. Peters (1989) Pan Books Ltd., Cavaye Place, London SW10 9PG.
Managing Change in Primary Care	M. Pringle, J. Bilhhu, M. Dornan and S. Head (1991) Radcliffe Medical Press Ltd., 15 Kings Meadow, Ferry Hinksey Road, Oxford OX2 0DP.
The Change Masters	Rosabeth Moss Kanter (1983) Unwin Hyman Ltd, 15–17 Broadwick St, London W1V 1FP
Managing change in general practice: A step by step guide	N. Speigal, E. Murphy, A. Kinmonth, F. Ross, J. Bain and R. Coates (1992) *British Medical Journal*, **304**: 231–4.

Managing Change in Organisations	C. A. Carnall (1990) Prentice Hall International (UK) Ltd, Campus 400, Haylands Avenue, Hemel Hempstead, Herts.

NHS MANAGEMENT

The New National Health Service Organisation and Management	Chris Ham (1991) Radcliffe Medical Press Ltd, 15 Kings Meadow, Ferry Hinskey Road, Oxford OX2 0DP.
Change and Innovation A Challenge for the NHS	Tony Turrell (1986) The Institute of Health, Services Management, 75 Portland Place, London, W1N 4AN.
The Changing Face of the National Health Service in the 1990s	Editor Peter Spurgeon (1990) Health Service Management Centre, Longman, Longman House, Burnt Mill, Harlow CM20 2JE.

PRACTICE GUIDELINES

Southampton Beating Heart Disease Primary Care Guidelines	Dr Peter J. White and Nicki Spiegal (Unpublished) Available from: Aldermoor Health Centre, Aldermoor Close, Southampton.

PRACTICE NURSING

The Nurse in Family Practice: Practice Nurses & Nurse Practitioners in Primary Health Care	Anne Bowling and Barbara Stilwell (Eds.) (1988) Scutari Press, London.
The Practice Nurse, Theory and Practice	Pauline Jeffree (Ed.) (1990) Chapman and Hall

The Practice Nurse Handbook	K. J. Bolden and B. A. Takle (1989), Blackwall Scientific Publications, Osney Mead, Oxford OX2 0EL.
Nutrition Matters for Practice Nurses. A Handbook on Dietary Advice for use in the Community	A. R. Leeds, P. Judd and B. Lewis (Eds.) (1990 McGraw Hill Book Company, McGraw Hill House, Shoppenhanger Road, Maidenhead SL6 2QL.

RESEARCH

Research Methods for General Practitioners	David Armstrong, Michael Calnan and John Grace (1990) Oxford University Press, Walton Street, Oxford OX2 6DP.
Research Methods for Nurses	W. B. Ackerman and P. R. Lohnes (1981) McGraw-Hill Book Company, McGraw-Hill House, Shoppenhanger Road, Maidenhead SL6 2QL.

REPORTS

Neighbourhood Nursing A Focus For Care	Department of Health and Social Security (1986) HMSO, London.
A Strategy for Nursing	Department of Health (1989) HMSO, London.
Community Care, Agenda for Action	Department of Health (1988) HMSO, London.
General Practice in the NHS: 1990 Contract	Department of Health (1989) HMSO, London.
Working for Patients	Department of Health (1989) HMSO, London.

Caring for People	Department of Health (1989) HMSO, London.
The Health of the Nation	Department of Health (1992) HMSO, London.
The Patient's Charter	Department of health (1992) HMSO, London.
The Citizen's Charter	Office of Public Service and Science (1991) CM 1599. HMSO, London.

SMOKING

Beating the Ladykillers Women and Smoking	Bobbie Jacobson (1988) Pluto Press Ltd, The Works, 105a Torriana Avenue, London NW5 3RX.
Helping Patients and Clients to Stop Smoking. Assessing the Effectiveness of the Nurse's Role	Jill Macleod Clark, Sally Kendall and Sheila Haverty (1987) Health Education Authority, Hamilton House, Mabledon Place, London WC1H 9TX.
Smoke Stop. Group Leader's Manual. A Practical Guide to Setting Up and Running a Self-Help Group	Liz Batten (1984). Department of Psychology, The University, Southampton SO9 5NH.

TEAMWORK

Act Pack Teamwork in Practice	K. Munrow, J. Muir, A. Niel and T. Schofield (1992) Radcliffe Medical Press Ltd., 15 Kings Meadow, Ferry Hinskey Road, Oxford OX2 0DP.
Effective Teambuilding	J. Adair (1990) Gower Publishing Company, Gower House, Croft Road, Aldershot, Hants GU11 3HR.

Management Teams: *Why They Succeed or Fail*	R. M. Belbin (1981) Heineman (William) Ltd., Micheline House, 81 Fulham Road, London SW3 6RB.
Developing Teamwork in Primary Health Care: A Practical Workbook	P. Pritchard and J. Pritchard (1992) Oxford University Press, Walton Street, Oxford OX2 6DP.
Primary Health Care Team Workshop Manual *A Guide to Planning and Managing Workshops for Primary Health Care Teams*	Health Education Authority (1991) Hamilton House, Mabledon Place, London WC1H 9TX.

TIME MANAGEMENT

How to Get Control of Your Time and Your Life	Allan Laken (1973) Gower Publishing Company, Croft Road, Aldershot Hants GU11 3HR.

QUALITY

The Definition of Quality and Approaches to its Assessment Vol 1	A. Donabedian (1980) Health Administration Press, Michigan, USA.
International Journal of Health Care Quality Assurance	*See* 'Useful journals'.
Quality Assurance in Health Care	*See* 'Useful journals'.
Managing for Quality in General Practice	Donald Irvine (1990) Kings Fund Centre, 126 Albert Street, London NW1 7NF.
Developing Quality in Health Education and Health Promotion	C. Totten (Ed.) (1992) Society of Health Education and Health Promotion Specialists, c/o Lisburn Health Centre, Linerhall Street, Lisburn, N. Ireland BT28 1LU.

DISTANCE LEARNING PACKS

CHD: Reducing the Risk (O.U. Pack)	T. Heller, L. Bailey, M. Gott and M. Howes (1987) Open University in association with the HEC. The Open University, Department of Health and Social Welfare, Centre for Continuing Education, Walton Hall, Milton Keynes MK7 6AA
Prevention in practice	G. Barnes, A. Freter, P. Hawclock, I. Koppel, G. Roberts, T. Schofield, N. Spiegal and J. Tudor Hart (1992)
Team-Working in Practice	K. Munro, J. Miur, A. Niel and T. Schofield (1992)
Cholesterol in Practice	P. Hunt and M. Lawrence (1992) All Published by Radcliffe Medical Press Ltd, 15, King's Meadow, Ferry Hinksey Road, Oxford OX2 0DP.
Health Promotion in Primary Health Care. An Open Learning Package for Practice Nurses.	Published by English National Board (1989) Victory House, 170 Tottenham Court Road, London W1P 0HA.

Useful names and addresses

HEA Primary Health Care Unit
The Churchill Hospital
Headington
Oxford OX3 7LJ

Tel: 0865-226059/60/61

National Facilitator
Development Project
HEA Primary Health Care Unit
The Churchill Hospital
Headington
Oxford OX3 7LJ

Tel: 0865-226035/36/52/53

Health Education Authority
Hamilton House
Mabledon Place
London WC1H 9TX

Tel: 071-383-3833

Royal College of Nursing
20 Cavendish Square
London W1M 0AB

Tel: 071-409-3333 (BT)
071-872-0840 (Mercury)

Association of Primary Care
Facilitators
Members Secretary
Janet Baker
Facilitator in Primary Care
Health Education Department
Hereford and Worcester
FHSDA
St Marys Hospital
Burghill
Hereford HR4 7RF

Tel: 0432-760324 ext 3309

United Kingdom Central
Council for Nursing,
Midwifery and Health Visiting
23 Portland Place
London W1N 3AF

Tel: 071-637-7181

Royal College of General
Practitioners
14 Princes Gate
Hyde Park
London SW7 1PU

Tel: 071-581-3232

Kings Fund Centre
126 Albert Street
London NW1 7NF

Tel: 071-267-6111

Eli Lilly National Clinical Audit
Centre
University of Leicester
School of Medicine
Leicester General Hospital
Gwendolen Road
Leicester LE5 4PW

Tel: 0533-584353

Local Health
Promotion/Education Unit
Full list of names and
addresses available from
Health Education Authority,
London.